SIMPLE GUIDE
TO USING
HERBAL MEDICINE

ABOUT THE AUTHOR

With a childhood history involving significant use of anti-biotics, then later in his twenties prescribed addictive tranquillisers as treatment for stress, which he successfully weaned himself off using natural methods, PHILIP EVANS counts himself very fortunate indeed to have 'discovered' Herbal Medicine some ten years later in 1986. He subsequently left the career path he was following and trained for four years as a medical herbalist, gaining his qualification as a Member of the National Institute of Medical Herbalists, the oldest body of professional herbalists in the world, which was founded in 1864.

A past Hon. General Secretary of the Institute, he has been practising in Kent since 1990, where he runs two busy Herbal Dispensaries open to the public, and is actively supporting the current moves towards the recognition and registration of qualified herbalists by the UK Department of Health.

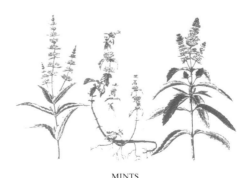

MINTS

Mentha viridis, Mentha pulegium, Mentha piperita

Herb illustrations – courtesy *A Modern Herbal* by Mrs M. Grieve, 1931

SIMPLE GUIDE
TO USING

HERBAL MEDICINE

PHILIP EVANS

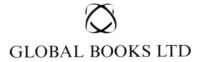

GLOBAL BOOKS LTD

Simple Guides • Series 4
NATURAL HEALTH

Simple Guide to Using
HERBAL MEDICINE
by Philip Evans

First Published 2001 by

GLOBAL BOOKS LTD
PO Box 219, Folkestone, Kent, England CT20 3LZ

© Global Books Ltd 2001

ISBN 1–86034–052–0

British Library Cataloguing in Publication Data
A CIP catalogue entry for this book
is available from the British Library

Set in Times New Roman 11 on 12pt by Mark Heslington, Scarborough, North Yorkshire
Printed in England by The Cromwell Press, Trowbridge, Wiltshire

Contents
•••••

Foreword
• • • • •

W hilst there are some excellent books on herbal medicine by well-qualified herbalists and eminent authorities on the subject, the authors tend to make too many assumptions about the reader's ability to derive and use information from them. Consequently, they serve as *introducers* or appetite-whetters to the subject of herbal medicine rather than becoming the useful handbooks they set out to be. Increasingly, the public is seeking practical support and informed discussion about *using* this form of natural treatment.

To date, no-one has really written a book exclusively from the point of view of the *user*, or would-be user, of herbal medicine, telling it as it is for *them*. As a result, many would-be users of herbal medicine remain confused in an environment of conflicting information, sometimes scaremongering, sometimes hope tinged with doubt.

This book, therefore, is intended to guide you through the maze that may confront you when you first start thinking of herbal medicine as a treatment for yourself or for those close to you.

☐

The reason for this confusion is simple: people. Herbal medicine treats people, not illnesses. You cannot say what herb you use for stomach ulcers, for instance; it depends on whose stomach ulcers you are talking about. There are twenty or more herbs that could be used for stomach ulcers in different people.

This is why people get confused, because they read a herbal book or an article in a newspaper or magazine, saying that this or that herb is good for migraines, or hot flushes, or irritable bowel, or which boosts the immune system, or whatever, and then become convinced that a particular herb is the one they should use.

We know this from the experience of our herbal dispensaries where people phone or visit asking such questions as 'What herb do you give for high blood pressure? Or eczema? Or depression? Or arthritis?' The answer usually has to be along the lines: 'Those herbs in the right quantities which suit that particular condition in that person. Therefore it would serve you best of all to see a qualified herbalist.'

Further confusion then arises because once people have been convinced they need a certain herb, they do not know how much of the herb to take, how often to take it, when to increase or decrease the dose, where to buy it, in what form to take it, how long to take it for, when to change it for a different herb or herbs, whether it may react with other medication they are taking, and so on.

They may also read a different article, or someone else may say that another herb is best for their condition, and so begins a long, often quite expensive, process of 'shooting in the dark', where people try this herb, then that herb, or a mixture of herbs, guessing at the dose, often for quite long periods and often to no avail. Where a herbal medicine does work when taken on a 'try-it-and-see' basis in this way, it is precisely because that herb is suited to the constitution and physiological imbalances of that person, and therefore it *is* the right herb for them.

The old saying 'one person's meat is another person's poison' certainly applies equally to herbal medicine as it does to diet, since the herb or herbs that are right for one person's arthritis, or irritable bowel, or allergies, or whatever, may be no use at all for another person's. This is because herbal medicine treats *people*, not illnesses or symptoms.

☐

So Echinacea, for instance, much-publicized over the past few years as the magic medicine for building up the immune system, may not be the best herb for building up the immune system of *all* people; other herbs may be more appropriate and other changes in life-style, diet, or drug use may be necessary. Herbs on their own cannot be expected to build up the immune system regardless of whatever the individual is doing to run it down in the first place.

So, too, with St John's Wort (*Hypericum perforatum*), which has also been at the forefront of the public's perception of herbal medicine in recent times, although it has been used by mankind for millenia. Much to professional herbalists' horror and dismay, it has been characterized as if it were an 'anti-depressant' that has just been discovered and that can replace drug anti-depressants as a direct alternative.

A professional herbalist would never call St John's Wort an anti-depressant, rather it is a herb that has, among other actions, a sedative, calming, and building effect on the nervous system, which in some cases (particularly where the nervous system has been hyperactive) but not all, can help people who are depressed.

St John's Wort does not suit all people who are depressed, however; some people actually need their nervous system stimulating at certain times rather than calming, and this is why it does not work for everyone who takes it as an 'anti-depressant'. Add to this the fact that it also has a number of other actions within the body, and that consequently there are a number of other conditions that herbalists would consider it for, and you can see why it is necessary to know what you are doing with St John's Wort before applying it in a blanket fashion to all people who are depressed.

Self-evidently, this is why it is invariably far better to consult a qualified herbalist about the use of St John's Wort, rather than just use it in a limited way, which does not do justice to the full capacity of this wonderful plant.

So, let us be clear, this guide does not set out to demonstrate that herbal medicine is the cure for all ills – far from it: there is a whole range of life-threatening emergencies and illnesses which can only be intercepted by modern pharmaceutical drugs or by surgery. This is not to say, however, that the use of herbal medicines even in this context is entirely without merit in a supportive role. Moreover, there is a whole range of medical conditions which herbal medicine can address very successfully indeed, which is the core focus of this book.

Undoubtedly, modern orthodox medical practice does not utilize the capabilities of herbal medicine to anything like the degree it warrants (and which increasing numbers of people would like to see), for everyday illnesses seen in everyday medical practice. The *Simple Guide to Herbal Medicine* sets out to redress this imbalance.

Finally, one thing is for sure: you should not just think of using herbal medicine as an alternative to drug medicine that you have to take for the rest of your life; if it works, if you get the right herbal formula for the condition that needs healing, and if you take any other life-style measures that are necessary, then you stand a chance of actually getting better, and if you do, you will not need any sort of medicine any more.

PHILIP EVANS, MNIMH
Canterbury, Autumn 2000

1
••••

What is Herbal Medicine?

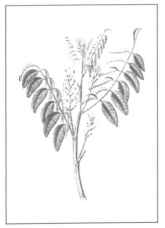

LIQUORICE
Glycyrrhina glabra

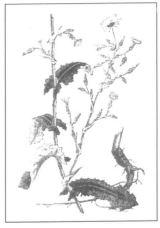

WILD LETTUCE
Lactuca virosa

'Do not consult holistic medicine if you are not prepared to change; for it may be in order to change that you became unwell in the first place'

H erbal Medicine is the system of medicine which uses plants in their whole and natural state to treat illness. The plants are made into various forms which include teas (or tisanes), tinctures, tablets, pills, powders, juices, waters, oils, creams, ointments, liniments, and poultices, which are then taken either internally (ingested), or applied to the body externally, as appropriate.

Herbal Medicine is not the same as Homeopathy, with which it is often confused; homeopathy uses very dilute forms of various substances, including derivatives which may be of herbal, mineral, or animal origin.

Herbal medicines are not necessarily safe just because they are natural; many plants are poisonous and therefore very dangerous. It requires a specialized knowledge of plants, a thorough understanding of their medicinal uses, and, in the case of people in 'Western' societies, not brought up with a cultural understanding of this nature, a proper training in order to be absolutely certain of their safe use.

Mankind has used herbal medicines for many thousands of years. Until very recently, the past three hundred years or so, they were the only type of medicines available to humanity.

Although it is often stated as if it were unquestionably so, it is not necessarily the case that modern people are healthier than before; indeed, there are many diseases nowadays that either did not exist or existed far less in the past, such as breast cancer, heart disease, irritable bowel syndrome, ME, and HIV/AIDS. We may be living longer, but this does not necessarily mean a greater degree of wellbeing or good health during our lives.

The increase in longevity is thought to be mainly because of an increase in hygiene, meaning that the burden of chronic (long-standing and sustained) infection on modern humans is reduced, compared to what our predecessors experienced. The word *healthy* should really be used to mean a state of true well-being (rather than mere longevity with no quality of life), which is indicated by having plenty of energy and stamina, a freedom from the symptoms of disease, good immunity to infections, and enthusiasm for one's future.

Many people instinctively feel an affinity towards herbal medicines as being natural and beneficial to mankind, even if they are not using them themselves, in much the same way that a good diet is considered beneficial to all people. In fact, herbal medicines are really an extension of the diet, to include plants with specific actions within the human body.

This natural enthusiasm for plant medicines probably stems from the knowledge that it is so ancient and therefore has been tried and tested successfully by all of our ancestors, being passed on to us precisely because it has proved to be of such worth throughout our history. Like good music, it has stood the test of time and would not have been passed down through the generations throughout the world if it were not a valuable and successful form of therapy.

Herbalists have always existed, and traditionally have been people with a detailed knowledge and understanding both of plant medicines and of illness (pathology), as well as possessing an understanding of and an empathy with people. In ancient societies many more people had a knowledge of herbal medicine because it was much more an integral part of their agricultural way of life than nowadays: we are really in the process of re-discovering herbal medicine for ourselves, having lost it, to a great extent, in Western societies until very recently after the advent and progress of medical science during the last three hundred years.

2
•••••

Philosophy of Herbal Medicine

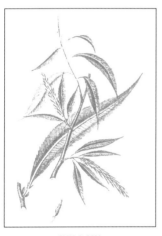

WILLOW
Salix alba

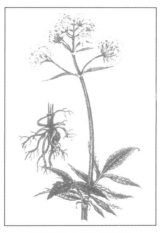

COMMON VALERIAN
Valeriana officinalis

UNDERSTANDING HUMAN PHYSIOLOGY

P hysiology means the way the body functions. Whereas modern science has brought about a tremendous increase in data concerning the functions of the body, the fact is that the human body has always functioned according to certain natural principles, whether or not mankind has understood it at any given point. So the thirteenth-century human body functioned along the same lines as the twentieth-century one, even though science had at that earlier time a very incomplete view of the details of bodily activity.

The very fact that new data keep emerging from the research and that analysis is continually being done by modern scientists, is in itself confirmation that science does not at any given point know all that there is to know about the human body.

Although a modern-day qualified medical herbalist or herbal practitioner in Western societies will generally have completed a four-year accredited training course to degree-level, with emphasis on both orthodox medical science and understanding of the therapeutic use of plants, and will have as complete an understanding of physiology and pathology as an orthodox-trained medical practitioner or doctor, it is not considered absolutely vital to have an in-depth knowledge of current physiology in order to successfully practise herbal medicine. This is because the traditional philosophy of herbal medicine encompasses many aspects of therapeutics that both in their success in analyzing and understanding ill-health and disease, and in their formulating of effective treatment strategies, are considerably in advance of current orthodox medical understanding of the nature of disease and the consequent steps for restoring health. We shall understand more about this as we go along.

In essence, the traditional way of perceiving and treating disease is generally termed 'holistic' (or 'wholistic') because it takes account of all aspects of the person's being, in other words the *whole* of the person, and explains why herbal medicine is often able to bring about successful healing where modern or orthodox medicine has been unsuccessful.

FUNDAMENTAL PRINCIPLES OF HERBAL MEDICINE

T he fundamental principles of herbal medicine are founded upon the premise that *the body heals itself, and knows what it is doing*. This is self-evidently true and experienced by all of us at different times in our lives. When we cut ourselves, for instance, there is an automatic function triggered within us that sets about the repair process; the blood congeals, white blood cells travel to the affected place in increased numbers, lymph activity increases there, pus forms, then a scab and finally a scar; these are not things we have to think about, they are automatic functions that take place within our bodies.

The pus and the scab and the scar may look ugly and may not be what we would have wanted, but they are Nature's way of clearing or healing the problem that was presented to the body. So also, when we eat something poisonous or contaminated like salmonella-infected food, we vomit and have diarrhoea. We do not have to think about it; we would not willingly choose to have diarrhoea but it is the body's automatic way of healing itself.

So, too, with all the functions within our wonderful human system: we do not have to think about the exchange of gases within the lungs, the peristalsis or movement within our intestine, the beating of our heart, the production of enzymes within the liver, these are all happening in nature's wonderful way automatically within us just because we are a part of nature's great whole. The body knows how to work and it knows what is best for it to do at any time. When we walk uphill the heart automatically beats faster in order to accommodate the extra energy required.

Why then, when we have an illness, or in particular when we experience the symptoms of an illness or ailment, should we think that something is going wrong and is not functioning as it should? Nature operating within the human body is not capable of carrying out something that should not be happening, it only ever carries out what is necessary at that time.

So when we have a headache, it is because the body needs to have a headache; perhaps the stress of too much work has raised the blood pressure and our body is trying to tell us something, in much the same way that when we touch a hotplate the pain in our hand tells us that we must withdraw it. When we have eczema why should we think that this should not be happening? If we have too much heat in our body then of course the body will put the heat out somewhere in the form of eczema or a rash; we should be asking what it is that we are doing that is making the body produce these symptoms, rather than decrying the fact that our body is producing the symptoms.

So, the fundamental premise of herbal medicine comes from the realization and acceptance that the body knows what it is doing and is always trying to heal itself, even if at first we cannot understand the details of this process.

3
•••••

How the Body Heals

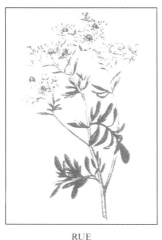

RUE
Ruta graveolens

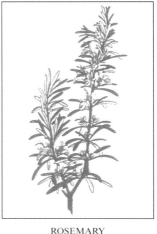

ROSEMARY
Rosmarinus officinalis

I t is worth looking at this healing process in a little more detail.

① All the parts of the body are related

This is clearly the case since the blood-stream contacts and links all tissues continuously. Therefore, we cannot deal with one part of the body without automatically needing to deal with all other parts of the body, since they are part of the one whole system. We cannot treat one part of the body without having an effect on the whole system. (This is, in fact, what gives rise to the side-effects of chemical drugs, as we shall see later.)

To illustrate this, if we benefit the liver during herbal treatment then all other parts of the body will benefit, since the blood, which is processed in the liver, will have a better quality which will be passed on to all the other organs and in turn to all parts of the body dependent on those organs. It is like a tree: if the nourishment and water supply are sound, then all parts of the whole tree will be sound. If our lungs work well and absorption of oxygen and vitality are sound, then this will equally benefit all other parts of the related whole.

Equally, if one part of the body is not working well, for instance the bowels, then this will be passed on to all other parts of the whole: in this case toxicity in the form of unwanted residues of food may well be re-absorbed and have a detrimental effect all through the system, perhaps leading to a person having a poor immunity because of toxicity deriving from a poor bowel function.

This point may be said to be the most striking difference between modern, orthodox Western medicine and traditional medicine: modern, orthodox medicine treats each symptom or ailment as if it were occurring in its own separated part of the body in isolation from other parts of the body, when in fact it is not separate at all, but is part of the whole body; a herbalist thinks of the body as a whole unit and treats the whole of it.

② There is a vitality in the body

This is not just a chemical process. This may be most graphically illustrated by the fact that when a body comes to the end of its life and the vitality leaves, we have what is termed death, despite all the chemical factors still being in place at that time; thus, there is a difference between a live body and a dead one, which is more than just the chemistry involved. In the same way some people, even for instance from the same family, have a lot more vitality or energy than others, despite the same genetic factors, diet, and environmental conditions, and this again reflects their own particular degree of tapping into this vital force or energy.

The word *energy* is the key here; and whereas modern orthodox science in general has recently embraced the view that everything in the universe is composed of energy or more specifically of differing rates of vibrations of one universal energy, the differing rates dictating the different forms of things that we see, rather than being, for instance, the simple solid forms which is what our senses report to us. Traditional medicine, especially the ancient Greek, Chinese and Ayurvedic (Indian subcontinent) medical philosophies, have always maintained (going back more than two thousand years), that everything is composed of energy.

Thus, understanding the flow of this energy within the human body, whilst knowing that the body itself is composed of this very energy – in common with all matter in the universe – and the way in which this relates to health and disease is an ancient concept and one which today, increasingly, is being accepted by orthodox science.

The energy flow, therefore, is fundamental to bringing about healing within the human body using herbal medicines, since herbal medicines themselves are also composed of this energy and as natural substances have a particular affinity or resonance with all other naturally-occurring substances, especially in this case the human body. We shall see more of this later.

③ Emotions affect the body

This is so basic a concept that it is amazing anyone could challenge it. Ask any woman whether her moods affect her menstrual periods, as well as the other way round; sometimes under great emotional stress a woman may stop having periods for months on end.

Equally, worrying too much can cause stomach ulcers, high blood pressure, worsen eczema, precipitate asthma, or cause tiredness. Prolonged anger affects the bile flow. The sight of a person holding a gun may make the adrenal glands produce more adrenaline which will flow around our bodies and increase our heart rate. A sudden shock can make the bowel evacuate itself completely, or the bladder empty its contents unannounced.

It is indeed surprising that modern orthodox medicine tends to treat only the body and not the emotions which have such an effect on the body overall. Where drugs *are* given for the emotions, this aspect or part of the person seems to be viewed in *isolation* from the physical part of them, and not as an integral part of the whole person.

Herbal medicine regards all aspects of the whole person as interactive, and thus it is often necessary to help both the patient's emotional state and their physical state as part of a successful treatment; when the emotions are harmonious the body works better; when the body works better the emotions benefit: it works both ways. This is a fundamental difference between the thinking of modern orthodox medicine and the ancient traditional forms of healing, such as herbal medicine, which have stood the test of time.

4
•••••

Diagnosis of the 'Whole Person'

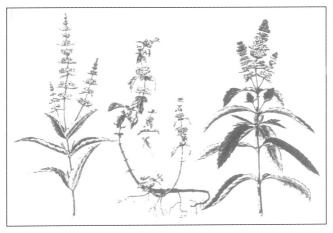

MINTS
Mentha viridis, Mentha pulegium, Mentha piperita

A t a consultation, there are some fundamental questions about the person that a herbalist will want answers to, but not necessarily by verbal questions and answers. This is why a consultation is required before a herbal prescription can be given, for it is a person who is being assessed for treatment, not a disease or disorder with a diagnostic label that is being treated without any interest in or insight into the person in question.

A herbalist will always want to know about the *whole* of a person's bodily functions. There are different ways in different herbal traditions for achieving this, again, not necessarily by verbal means. For instance, traditional Chinese medical practitioners tend to use non-verbal means of diagnosis such as observation of the abdomen, touch, palpation, and tongue- and pulse-analysis much more so than is practised in traditional Western herbal medicine. Western practice tends to use the verbal means of gathering information as well as some more common techniques of physical examination such as the taking of blood pressure.

The fundamental questions a herbalist will want answered may be summarized as follows:

- **Is the patient hot (or warm), or cold (cool)?**
  This is really the most fundamental of all the questions because from it so much information may be derived. Heat indicates over-activity in the functions of the organs. This is reflected in the increase in blood heat as the body tries to clear the heat generated by the overactivity away and out of the body via the blood to the skin and into the atmosphere.

  Coldness, on the other hand, indicates under-activity in the functions of the organs. This is reflected in the lack of heat in the blood as the body directs the heat out of the bloodstream into the organs to try to increase their dynamic functions.

The term 'homeostasis' is used in orthodox medicine to indicate the body's built-in tendency to adjust its own activities, such as its state of heat and coldness, in an endeavour to produce a state of balance where there is neither too much nor too little going on. The analysis given above is an example of exactly this taking place.

To the herbalist it is vital to know whether a person feels the heat, or the cold, or both, or feels too hot or too cold for no reason, since from this simple piece of information so much is indicated about the way their body is functioning. Equally, a lot of information may be gathered by observation (red face, white fingers, and so on), and by touch (cold or warm hands). All these apparently simple means of information-gathering are in fact fundamental diagnostic tools, and pave the way for successful treatment, as we shall see later on.

If the patient is too hot, they need cooling down; if too cold, they need warming up, since this is in fact what their own body is trying to do for itself; herbal medicines encourage and assist this natural process.

● **Is the patient damp (wet, clammy), or dry?**
This shows up most obviously in the skin (general dryness or clamminess, including a degree of sweating and any nervous sweat), but can also be ascertained by whether the bowel motions are too loose (diarrhoea) or too firm (constipated), whether there is catarrh, mucus or phlegm in the respiratory system (which are signs of dampness), and the nature of the urine flow (excessive flow shows dampness, reluctant flow shows dryness).

Whether the patient is damp or dry is an important sign because dampness shows there is too much moisture in the system which the body has to rid itself of, whilst dryness means that the body is having to hang on to all the moisture there is.

Since these four governing principles of heat, cold, dampness and dryness indicate how the body is functioning at this fundamental level which is so important to the assessment of a person's physiology, we may sum up the balance that exists between these four principles as follows:

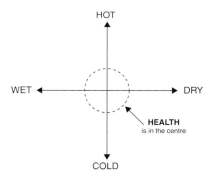

What change in diet, if any, the herbalist may well ask, does this person need to make to assist balanced functioning within their own system?

Since the energy of people can manifest in their body being either too hot or too cold, too damp or too dry, and since foods can also be classified as having an energy that is hot, cold, wet, or dry, it follows that food may be used as a tool to adjust the physiology of a person whose body is out of balance.

'Hot' and 'Cold' Food

The point about 'hot' and 'cold' foods is not whether they are heated up in terms of their temperature or cooled down as in refrigerated, or to whether they are in juicy sauces or in dry and crumbly form, but refers to the energy carried by the food. For instance, spices are generally hot whether they are heated up or not, cow's milk is very damp whether it is freeze-dried and consumed as a powder or simply drunk on its own.

Such treatment may be called the use of the 'energetics of food' and is not the same as dieting or any other form of food restriction, rather it emphasizes the use of certain foods for certain individuals whilst restricting the use of other foods, according to that person's constitution and any imbalances in their physiology.

We are reminded of Hippocrates' axiom: 'Let your food be your medicine and your medicine be your food.'

● **Which organs in the body are not functioning correctly?**
In natural therapy talk we often hear the expression 'balanced' in relation to the functions of the body, or that this or that organ is 'out of balance'. But what precisely does this mean? It is very important to understand what it means, since this is the basic precept or starting point of natural therapies, including herbal medicine. 'Balanced' means in fact that the organ in question is functioning neither too much nor too little, but just to the right degree, since either of these two extremes is not as it should be and therefore the organ will be 'out of balance': for

instance, in the case of the liver if there is too much activity, then too much bile may be produced and this may have consequences for the health of the bowel and consequently the body as a whole; if there is too little activity then there may not be enough bile and this, too, may have consequences for the digestion of food and for the body as a whole.

If the adrenal glands 'out of balance' then there may be an excessive production of adrenaline and the blood pressure may go up; if this situation is maintained for too long then it may result in the adrenal glands 'having a rest', the result of which may be sustained tiredness and low blood pressure, in fact, as the body seeks automatically to establish the state of balance or homeostasis we talked about before, by enforcing a state where the body may rebalance itself and move away from the overactivity originally causing the problem.

● **What emotions are contributing to the state of the organs?**

Ancient medical systems do not separate the emotions from the physical body, rather they are seen as part of a whole person, who has both physical and emotional aspects. Thus a herbalist will often end up discussing emotional issues with a patient. This in itself can be extremely helpful, and it frequently happens that the patient finds their own emotional healing through such a discussion, people often knowing precisely what their own problems are when given the chance to formulate their thoughts on the subject.

This is carried one stage further in traditional Chinese medicine, where there is said to be a direct link between certain major emotions and specific organs in the body. This is best illustrated by the diagram below:

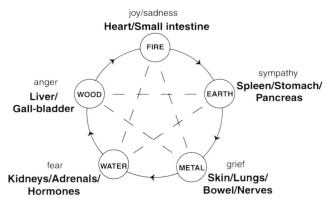

THE FIVE ELEMENTS

- **Which herbs are relevant to this person?**
  During the assessment the herbalist will be figuring out which organs are out of balance and therefore which herbs are relevant to the person, since different herbs 'target' different organs and either increase their function or decrease it.

  This will result in an individualized prescription for each person according to their own constitution and state of bodily function, *not* in the same standardized prescription for everyone who is depressed, or who has irritable bowel, or eczema, and as we shall see later, it may be either a very simple prescription containing only one herb, or quite a complicated formula or prescription containing many herbs.

5
• • • • •

Thinking About Using
Herbal Medicine

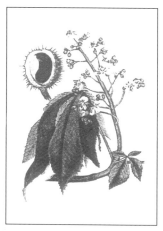

HORSE CHESTNUT
Æsculus hippocastanum

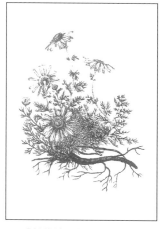

COMMON CHAMOMILE
Anthemis nobilis

M ore often than not, we find ourselves thinking about herbal medicine because someone else has put the idea in our mind. This person might be a friend, relative, or acquaintance during a discussion on illness in general, on another person's illness, or on that person's specific illness. It might be the author of a book, magazine or newspaper article that we have read, or something on a TV or radio programme. It might be seeing a shop selling health foods and 'herbal remedies', an article or advertisement selling herbal or health products. Or someone may simply recommend a herbal product or a particular therapist that has been helpful to them.

It is always good to have a recommendation for any product or service that we think of using. It reassures us and makes us feel more secure when someone else has already tried something and been pleased with it before us, whether it be a restaurant, a clothes shop or a garage.

When there has been no recommendation, however, we have to use our own judgement and initiative, and this seems to work along definite lines in the case of using herbal medicine.

The following thoughts and questions are likely to enter a person's mind when wishing to consider using herbal medicine:

- Do I grow medicines myself, as they are plants?
- Can I buy herbal medicines anywhere, or are they difficult to get?
- How do I find out where to buy them?
- How much will it cost, is it very expensive?
- How much do I take and for how long?
- What sort of medicines are there available? Are there tablets, liquids, or what?
- Do I have to tell my doctor?
- Will my doctor know where I can go to get them?

- Does my doctor use herbal medicines for his patients?
- Are they covered on the state-funded health scheme?
- What if they are poisonous or dangerous?
- Surely there must be people who know about or specialize in herbal medicine to help me through this process?

Such questions are common enough and have been put to the author many times by patients over the years. It is both odd and interesting that the last stage in the train of thought seems to be to try and find someone who is a professional in the field of herbal medicine, in other words, a herbalist.

Could it be that herbalists are not making their presence felt sufficiently, so that few people realize that there are indeed – certainly in the UK and other English-speaking countries – professional, well-trained, qualified herbalists that may be consulted?

The options available to the person wishing to use herbal medicine may be summed up as follows:

① Grow your own herbs and self-medicate. This has to be done with great care since many plants are poisonous. The choice of herbs, their doses, and the length of treatment, are factors that will have to be assessed for oneself.

② Go to a health food shop or another outlet selling herbal products and try buying herbs over-the-counter in various forms such as dried herbs, creams, tinctures, tablets, oils, ointments, juices, etc. following the *generalized* instructions on the label which are not specific to any *individual's* particular needs.

The choice of herb or herbs is another area of difficulty since there are *many* herbs that can be used for similar conditions. It is difficult for such an outlet to provide follow-up support since this sort of transaction is essentially a voluntary act on the part of the user, and not something that the outlet participates in other than as the supplier of a product which the user then uses at their own discretion.

③ Visit a qualified herbalist and get an individual prescription for your case, usually including a package of individualized dietary and other advice, and proper guidance throughout your treatment, however long it may or may not be, with follow-up care and the possibility of discussing your case with your practitioner as it progresses.

As will be seen from the case histories (Chapter 9), the correct handling of a case and the adjustment of a herbal prescription, which may contain from one to a dozen or more different herbs in differing doses, is something that can only be done on a individualized basis, since every person is unique.

Herbalists *cannot guarantee to help in all cases*, and any herbalist claiming to do so is to be avoided.

In fairness to lack of successes by herbalists, however, it should be pointed out that it is far easier to treat a person *before* their body has been subjected to the suppressive effects of drug medicines on their bodies, rather than *after* what may be several years of the use of these types of treatment on their systems.

Herbalists often have to work with the patient to get them off drug medicines before there is any possibility of the herbal medicines working to help their own bodies to function better for themselves, and this can sometimes prove difficult, and even impossible.

Qualified herbalists know under what circumstances it is best to work together with the drug medication being taken by a patient, rather than trying to get the herbal medicine to replace it.

6
•••••

Seeing a Herbalist

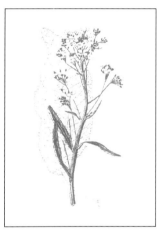 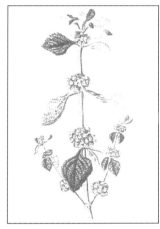

HORSERADISH
Cochlearia armoracia

WHITE HOREHOUND
Marrubium vulgare

QUALIFICATIONS

I n the UK at the time of writing it is not necessary for a practitioner to be professionally qualified *in any way* in order to practise as a herbalist – the right to practise being made possible under common law. In other English-speaking countries differing legislation is either in place or under way, some of it preserving the right for traditional practitioners to continue doing what they and their ancestors have always done in continuing to use herbal medicines.

In some European countries, including France, Italy, Spain and Portugal, it is an offence for anyone other than a state-licensed doctor to prescribe herbal medicines, and an offence for anyone other than a state-registered pharmacist to sell herbal products.

A mistake that orthodox doctors often make is in elevating their own medical training in their thinking to a position of superiority over that of any practitioner of natural medicine, including a qualified herbalist. This position tends to encourage a negative, sometimes dismissive, attitude in their approach to herbalists and herbal medicine.

In fact, nothing could be further from the truth, since the medical training undergone by a qualified herbalist (in the UK over four years) leads to a Degree (BSc) in Herbal Medicine available at four universities. It is equivalent to the qualification held by a doctor, whilst being far wider since it also covers the use of medicinal plants and the profound philosophy underlying their successful use in practice.

There are currently strong moves in the UK towards carrying through the status of properly qualified herbalists to that of an officially-recognized profession, which would both ensure the right of qualified herbalists to practise and at the same time safeguard the public from the possible dangers of an unregulated market in herbal medicines.

It is a tricky question because after all, herbs are nature's gift to the whole of humanity, and people should at all times in the future be free, as they have been in the past, to use them as their choice of medicines in a relatively unrestricted manner if they so wish.

Seeing a practitioner, however, may be viewed as something different, because if someone sets themselves up as a herbalist and charges money for their services, then the public is equally entitled to know that the practitioner is educated and properly trained in their profession, and safe in what they do.

Details of the main professional bodies to which qualified herbalists belong, as well as the major institutions offering training in herbal medicine, are given in the *Appendix*.

CONSULTATIONS

T he advantage of seeing a qualified herbalist who is a member of a recognized professional body is that she or he will be properly trained and experienced, and will also follow a code of practice and have professional insurance – all for the benefit and safeguarding of the patient.

One of the main differences people often remark on at a herbal consultation is how helpful and pleasant it is for them to have time to talk about themselves and about *all* their ailments. This is because, as we have seen, the herbalist takes a holistic approach, seeing the body as an integrated whole.

In general medical practice, on the other hand, doctors often have to see thirty to fifty patients per day; under these circumstances, of course, time has to be restricted or rationed, and patients inevitably feel under pressure to be quick and not to use up the doctor's time, often reporting that they feel their own ailments are trivial compared to others on the doctor's list.

Equally, one can see how under this sort of time pressure it is the symptoms and not the root causes of ailments that have to be addressed, since there is no time to delve into the root causes. Doctors themselves will acknowledge that they only treat the symptoms of illnesses and do not search for the underlying cause. For instance, they give antacids for indigestion rather than go into the patient's diet, which might reveal the reason for the excessive stomach acid, but which would take more time and a greater understanding.

However, whereas patients are often incredibly understanding of the doctor's dilemma in having to try and operate under these constraints of time, and often fully appreciate the pressure the doctor is under – thereby attributing the doctor's failure to sort out their problem to a lack of time – there is, surely, a more profound reason for this problem.

The fact is *too many people are not getting better*. If they were, they would not have to keep going back to see the doctor, the doctor would not be so busy, and there would be more time for proper in-depth consultations by doctors.

So, orthodox medicine has perhaps created its own self-perpetuating problem: precisely because it only treats the symptoms of illnesses and not the root causes, people do not get better in sufficient numbers, so they have to keep going back to the doctor, thus restricting the doctor's time and ensuring that the root cause cannot be unveiled, which keeps the problem recurring over and over again.

The problem is made that much greater because few orthodox practitioners are properly informed about diet or the human physiology as a whole.

So it is that in herbal practice one of the most noticeable things patients find is that there is time to gain an in-depth understanding of the illness, and time to discuss all the symptoms within the body. This is very important of course since the body works as a united whole, not as a series of unrelated parts. It needs to be regarded, understood, and treated as such, if a natural medicine, which will allow the body's own healing processes to come through, is to be successful.

PATIENT–PRACTITIONER RELATIONSHIP

I n herbal practice the relationship of the patient to the practitioner is considered very important; in particular the herbalist must have an affinity for and an interest in *people* in order to be able to relate to *all* the aspects of the patient as a person, not just as a body presenting symptoms.

The herbalist must understand, as must any good doctor, that this is a person in front of her or him, with many aspects, both in the material and the emotional sense.

In order to be a good herbalist, therefore, it is *not* enough merely to have an academic understanding of the subjects of medical science. Anatomy, physiology, pathology, diagnosis and theoretical treatment strategies do indeed form part of the understanding possessed by a capable herbalist, but this is also balanced by an understanding of the subtleties of human nature. This makes it possible for the treatment to be tailored correctly to match that unique individual with all of her or his idiosyncrasies.

☐

At this point it may be of interest to point out that the third most common complaint by patients regarding their doctor is that he/she does or did not pay sufficient attention to them *as a person*, preferring instead to generalize about their condition ('It's irritable bowel, people have to live with it'). Or, instead being engrossed in the computer on his desk rather than engaging the patient in eye-contact in the way that is normal between human beings.

Equally, patients are often very willing to forgive even gross deficiencies on the part of their doctor (such as incorrect diagnoses, failure to properly monitor conditions such as high blood pressure, failure to pick up drug side-effects that the patient has complained of), when the doctor looks after the patient as a *human being*. If this human dimension does exist and they relate well to him/her there is clearly an opportunity for best practice to flourish – thereby underlining just what an important aspect of health-care the patient–physician relationship is. Patients will often defend their doctor's errors of judgement to a surprising degree if they get on well with him/her as a person.

Once a good and fair mutual relationship has been established, therefore, between patient and practitioner, the 'chemistry' of the patient's healing may begin to take place on a sure foundation.

7

∙ ∙ ∙ ∙ ∙

Herbal Treatments

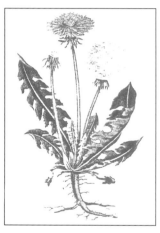

DANDELION
Taraxacum officinale

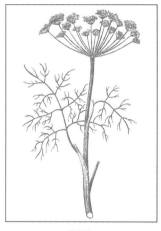

DILL
Peucedanum graveolens

Comparison between the treatments by orthodox medicine and by herbal medicine of the six most common illnesses seen in herbal practice.

T he first of the two commonest complaints on the part of patients is that they are rarely offered any alternative by their doctor when they consult him over a medical condition; all that they are offered as a matter of routine is orthodox or drug medicine.

The second commonest complaint heard is that the patient does not merely want to have the *symptoms* of a condition treated, which as doctors themselves will admit is what drug medicine does, they actually want to have the root cause of their problem found and dealt with, so that their own body may heal itself up, once this root cause has been properly addressed.

This latter course – of wanting to find, and then dealing with, the root cause in terms of what is not functioning properly in the patients's body – is exactly what herbal medicine under the supervision of a qualified herbalist will seek to do.

It may therefore be of interest to analyse the treatment of six of the illnesses most commonly seen by qualified herbalists, and to compare these treatment approaches with those adopted by orthodox or drug medicine, in order to highlight the differences between the two. This may in itself go some way towards explaining the frequent success of herbal medicine in dealing with these particular illnesses which drug medicine often finds extremely difficult to resolve successfully or to the patient's satisfaction.

1   ECZEMA

ORTHODOX DRUG TREATMENT   Treats the symptoms alone by using creams of various types: moisturising creams; antibiotic creams (if required); increasingly strong steroid (hydrocortisone) creams if necessary as the treatment continues; emollient oils for baths; emollient hairwashes.

HERBAL TREATMENT   Regards eczema, along with many other types of inflammatory (red, hot, usually itchy) skin conditions, as a sign of too much *heat* within the person's body; therefore the aim of treatment is to reduce the person's body heat (which is borne in the blood). Very often this is caused in part by the diet, and it is therefore necessary for the sufferer to remove from the diet those foods which may be unsuitable to her or his physiology, thereby causing a form of toxicity and resultant heat.

If the organs of elimination (liver, bowels, kidneys) are not working well enough, then the toxicity and heat may not be dealt with, and so the heat will have to come out through another means (the skin): this is what we call eczema. There are other forms of toxicity too, such as environmental pollution, food pollution (pesticide residues, etc), which should be dealt with by the organs of elimination in the person's body, but if these organs are deficient in their function then these factors may have an effect that they would not have otherwise.

The adrenal glands play a large role in the reduction of heat by producing natural steroids (anti-inflammatory hormones) within the human body, and their function often needs to be improved. The reason that stress is often a factor in the onset of eczema is that it reduces the body's capacity to produce these natural steroids, as the adrenal glands are too engaged in producing adrenaline in response to the stress.

It is more difficult to treat eczema when the patient has been using steroid (hydrocortisone) creams, because they are what is known as a *suppressive* treatment. By doing the body's own work for it, these creams make the person's own production of natural steroids go dormant, thus making it difficult for the natural anti-inflammatory processes to function at all.

Typically, this approach worsens the condition by driving it deeper inwards (suppressing it), whereas the body itself was trying to drive the heat outwards through the skin.

Consequently, this increases the body's attempts to rid itself of the heat and in effect increases the eczema. The result is that stronger and stronger steroid creams have to be prescribed by doctors, a situation very often seen in herbal practice. When a patient stops using a steroid cream their own body often finds it very difficult to deal with the heat at all, as the result of the suppressive effect of the steroids, and the eczema naturally worsens, meaning that ever-stronger steroid creams may well have to be prescribed. This is a 'vicious circle' where the body has in effect become reliant on the steroid cream to do its own job for it, and then cannot do without it.

This is not the same as a 'healing crisis', which can occur in the treatment of eczema (and in other conditions too) using herbal medicine. A healing crisis means that the correct therapeutic steps are being taken, by either diet changes or herbal treatment, or both, to finally let the body do what it has been trying to do all the time, which is to rid itself of the excess heat. Thus, in the same way that eczema itself should be seen as the body's attempt to rid itself of excess heat, and therefore a 'good' thing if we want to call it anything, so a healing crisis should be seen as a 'good' thing, too, since it indicates that the body is responding to the treatment and ridding itself most definitely of the heat that is the problem, thus causing the 'worsening' of the symptoms.

Changing the diet appropriately can take the pressure off the digestive system and allow a respite in which those organs in the body responsible for the reduction of toxicity and heat (the liver, the bowel, the kidneys, and the adrenal glands) can begin working better since there is less for them to have to deal with. Equally, the use of the correct herbs for that person to increase the elimination of heat through the liver, the bowel, and the kidneys will assist in the reduction of blood-borne heat throughout the system. At the same time, the restoration of the functioning of the adrenal glands and reduction of any stress by the appropriate herbs will enable the person's own body to cope once more with excesses in the body's heat should they reappear once again.

Externally, creams may be given to reduce inflammation locally and to deal with any infection in the eczema. Bathing herbs may also be used as washes or, especially in the case of babies, as a means of administering the herbal medicine through absorption via the skin during bathtime.

No herbalist can guarantee a cure for eczema in every case, but skin problems in general are one of the areas where herbal medicine has a very high success rate, largely because, in contrast to orthodox medicine, it takes a profound viewpoint of the origin of the condition within the sufferer's body, and takes measures to rectify the *cause* and not just treat the symptoms.

2   IRRITABLE BOWEL SYNDROME (IBS)

ORTHODOX DRUG TREATMENT The diagnosis 'IBS' is usually given by doctors when there is no other diagnostic label that can be given, frequently following many investigations and tests which have proved negative, and is therefore really a diagnostic term by default, there being no other term that can be applied. Doctors often attribute IBS to stress, and people are told they are stressed even if they do not feel they are, and that this is the cause of the problem. They are told to eat more fibre, even if they already do eat a lot, but are seldom asked any further questions about their diet or given any further advice on it, which is strange since a digestive condition is obviously likely to be related to diet. They are often told that they will have to live with it since there is nothing that can be done about the condition. Sometimes patients are given anti-diarrhoeal drugs, bulk laxatives containing gel, or anti-spasmodic drugs.

HERBAL TREATMENT Herbalists will almost always want to begin their questions by asking about the patient's diet. They do not regard IBS as a single condition, but rather one that will be an individual one in every patient's case, and so will require an individual approach in each case; for instance, some people have predominantly diarrhoea, while others are constipated; there is often a considerable amount of abdominal bloating, and often pain of varying intensity and type.

Dietary changes suggested by a herbalist will be tailored to the individual's constitution and the nature of their bowel movements, for instance it is inappropriate in many cases for someone with diarrhoea to eat more fibre, since this is quite likely to make the loose bowel motions worse.

Whilst it is not possible to generalize about the appropriate diet to follow in order to allow the healing of the bowel in IBS – some people finding that a cow's milk-free diet is really helpful, others that a wheat-free diet proves successful – nonetheless, it is true to say that in a large percentage of cases herbalists find that *yeast* is the offending problem. All too often the bowel has too high a content of yeast or *Candida albicans* (the name of the human intestinal yeast), and reduction of this level by the appropriate change of diet will in many cases bring about a great improvement.

Since yeast in a warm, enclosed space in the presence of sugar and food matter sets up a fermentation process and produces alcohol (like a miniature brewery!), and expands causing a lot of gas, it is easy to see how this could cause the symptoms of irritable bowel. The inflammation caused by such overactivity of the yeast is what produces the changes in bowel motions. Whether there is too much yeast in the bowel *for that person* is very easy to ascertain, by asking whether the person has or is prone to either thrush or athlete's foot (both of which are fungal infections), or is allergic to penicillin (a fungus or yeast).

If the answer to any of these questions is yes, then it is likely that a yeast reduction diet will bring results. Additionally, from the case history it will often be found that the onset of IBS was closely related in time to the starting of hormone replacement therapy (HRT) or the taking of the contraceptive Pill (both of which often cause thrush and are therefore likely to have increased the person's intestinal and systemic yeast level). This goes some way to explaining why four times more women suffer from IBS than men.

Furthermore, in the person's history it will frequently be found that there has been a spell of multiple and heavy administration of antibiotics, for instance over the course of one to three years, often at school age for such conditions as repetitive tonsillitis, glue ear, or cystitis. Whilst these antibiotics do a job in killing off the infection at the time, they weaken the immune system and make it more likely the infection will return, thus necessitating more antibiotics, and so on in a vicious circle. Also, antibiotics often cause thrush, and in the case of many people their immune system does not completely recover from this immune deficit and the yeast problem remains, often re-emerging in adult life when the conditions all add up to what doctors call irritable bowel syndrome, but which is actually in these cases, at least, a problem of yeast-excess.

Finally, IBS is evidently a modern condition, there being no real record of it having existed, and certainly not to the degree and extent it does nowadays, before the advent of artificial hormones and antibiotics. This, too, lends weight to its origin in man-made drugs.

□

The emphasis in using herbs to treat irritable bowel syndrome if it is a Candida (yeast) problem, is on herbs which will restore the immune system as well as improving the whole digestive system's functioning. This can enable the bowel to regain its proper functioning too. Since the digestive system is a continuous unit from the mouth to the anus, attention will be paid to all parts of it from the proper production of saliva onwards, and including the several organs that compose the whole system, not just regarding the lower part (the bowel) as a separate and isolated bit of it.

Thus, herbs for the improvement of the functioning of the stomach, the pancreas, duodenum, and liver may all need to be included, depending on the individual case.

Any element of stress will also be dealt with by the appropriate herbs to either calm or restore the nervous system; this often manifests in the nature of the pain, usually as sharp or spasm pain, since the bowel is very responsive to the emotions. The pain is often the result of the bloating, however, and when this begins to subside the pain does too.

Often, people feel better after only two or three weeks of the correct advice and treatment, and frequently report a great improvement in overall well-being, energy, and mood as this troublesome condition begins to heal up.

3 HORMONAL PROBLEMS

ORTHODOX DRUG TREATMENT Before the advent in
the 1960s of the contraceptive Pill in its many combinations
of the two major female hormones (oestrogen and
progesterone), and later of Hormone Replacement Therapy
(HRT) in its different forms, orthodox or drug medicine
really had little to offer in the way of treatment for women
experiencing hormonal imbalances, meaning either deficit or
excess of the main hormones progesterone and oestrogen.
Clearly, it is by no means surprising that the advent of these
two types of drugs revolutionized the treatment of female
hormonal problems, and nowadays doctors freely prescribe
one or other of these drugs for all types of hormonal
conditions. If these hormonal treatments are not successful,
then recourse is often eventually made to operative
measures, including total or partial hysterectomy.

Apart from the fact that determining the correct
proportions of hormone for each individual is often very
difficult to achieve, one of the main problems with this is
that the drugs themselves can so severely interfere with other
processes in the female body. There are many possible side-
effects, some of them very serious, and these side-effects are
a common problem seen in herbal practice.

HERBAL TREATMENT Herbalists, on the other hand, have
always had a considerable storehouse of medicines available for
female hormonal problems. The major difference between
orthodox drugs used by doctors and natural medicines used by
herbalists is that whereas drugs artificially put into the body the
hormones which the person's own body is not producing on its
own, herbal medicine encourages the person's own body to
produce the right amount of hormone *for itself* by means of
gentle stimulation or regulation of the pituitary, thyroid and
adrenal glands as well as the ovaries.

It is, therefore, no longer a question of striving to find the right
hormones to put *into* the person's body in an artificial way,
(including the use of 'natural hormonal creams' currently on

the market), but rather of encouraging her own body to produce the right balance of progesterone and oestrogen for itself.

Such a process can be difficult and take many months of treatment, especially when the problem goes back many years; it is made more difficult again when the patient has been taking artificial hormones since they *suppress* the body's own ability to produce the correct balance of hormones for itself – the ovaries, in particular, going dormant under the effect of artificial hormones, and they then have to 'wake up again' when these are stopped and herbal treatment is started.

Both in principle, however, and in practice, hormonal problems such as irregular periods, heavy periods, PMS (Pre-Menstrual Syndrome) including mood changes and fluid retention, fibroids, polycystic ovaries, endometriosis, hot sweats, palpitations, and cyclic moodiness can be treated and helped using the correct herbal medicines for the individual concerned.

The heat present in the female body during the menopause often needs to be corrected using dietary changes also. The moods, as any woman knows well, are inextricably tied up with hormones, so herbalists do not treat any mood changes as a separate entity on their own, but rather as part of the whole picture of the person when the hormones are out of balance.

The 'menopause' has acquired a meaning currently as if it is inevitable that a woman will feel stressed, moody, anxious, hot, depressed, and experience sweats, palpitations, and many other symptoms, when her periods begin to stop, but the word itself just means 'stopping of the periods'. If the hormones are in correct balance, there will be no symptoms at all, just a natural cessation of the periods, as evidenced by the fact that many women do stop their periods without any unpleasant symptoms: these are the people whose hormones are naturally in balance.

Where a herbal treatment works, it will indeed be the woman's own body that is working better, *assisted* by the herbal medicine, not the herbal medicine that is 'making' it do so in an artificial way. For this reason, once the woman's body has acquired the habit of working well for itself again, then herbal medicine will no longer be necessary – quite unlike drug hormones which, often enough, women do have to take for very long periods of time.

4 HEADACHES AND MIGRAINES

ORTHODOX DRUG TREATMENT   Doctors, quite rightly, frequently send patients for further tests in cases of repetitive head pain, where their own investigations, such as checking of blood pressure, have proved fruitless. Where these prove clear, and if there is a neck problem which could be leading to the head pain some doctors will suggest treatment by a chiropractor, osteopath, or physiotherapist. Some doctors will suggest avoiding the classic four foods for migraine: cheese, chocolate, coffee, and red wine.

Often, doctors diagnose stress as the cause of the headaches, and suggest a holiday. Some doctors will recommend relaxation strategies. Most often, however, the patient is told that the pain is something that some people get, and painkillers of various types are prescribed, some of which can be addictive, or the patient continues to take their own over-the-counter painkillers.

HERBAL TREATMENT   A herbalist will want to get to the root cause of the head pain problem. This can often be a drug side-effect, something which doctors frequently seem to be unaware of, or choose to overlook the possibility that it could be a factor.

A herbalist will investigate the possibility of foods causing headaches. The four classic foods mentioned above all contain substances that are basically stimulants. Where the person's body tends to become over-stimulated in any case, avoiding these four can really be successful.

There is more to food intolerance than this, however, and a herbalist will know how to ask the correct questions to cast more light on this possibility.

Head pain is essentially caused by a *blockage* in the flow of energy to the head: this can happen because of a *mechanical* disturbance (such as a trapped nerve in the neck), or because of a *functional* disturbance, meaning that the functions of the body are disturbed. For instance, when there is too much tension in the muscles, the small arteries in the head become constricted (vasoconstriction); the body will attempt to counterbalance this by expanding the arteries so that the blood can get through them properly again (vasodilation). This increase in blood flow is what can cause a pounding headache or migraine.

So we have a problem of tension having a physiological knock-on effect resulting in head pain: by treating the root cause, which is the tension or overactivity in the muscles, the blood flow becomes normal and the end result, the pain, no longer occurs.

Herbalists may also suggest relaxation methods and techniques by which patients can help themselves, and many patients are keen to learn such methods by attending classes such as yoga or meditation.

In herbal treatment, it is impossible to say which herbs should be given for head pain, as each individual case needs to be treated as a unique individual. But attention is given to all systems in the person's body, not just the head itself or the nervous system. It may be necessary, therefore, to give herbs for the digestive system, in order to relieve congestion either in the bowels or liver, for instance, which are often connected to head pain, and can show up as the nausea associated especially with migraine.

The blood pressure may be raised, and therefore herbs for the nervous system will be called for, especially those which act on the vagus nerve and calm the autonomic branch of the nervous system. Once again, it is a question of treating the physiological imbalances within the person suffering with head pain, of treating the root cause within her or his body, and not just treating the end result or symptom, which is the pain itself.

5   ALLERGIES AND SENSITIVITIES

ORTHODOX DRUG TREATMENT   Specific allergy testing is seldom done by doctors in general practice because there is no consensus on their being any absolutely accurate method of testing. The old method of 'patch-testing' on the skin, which many patients think of asking for, is seldom done nowadays as it proved to be dangerous for some people in the case of severe allergy.

Patients are often told, following a blood test, that they have an allergy (due to raised antibody levels), but that they must find out for themselves what it is. Methods of allergy testing for specific substances include an 'in vitro' (laboratory) blood test now available. Treatments for all types of allergies by orthodox medicine are usually limited nowadays to oral antihistamines, and sprays (including steroid sprays) to treat the symptoms of the allergy. Treatment in allergic emergencies is given by antihistamine and adrenaline injections.

HERBAL TREATMENT   The question of whether they have an allergy is one that more and more people are asking themselves when they have symptoms of various types that will not respond to treatment. Allergy will affect either the skin (e.g. rashes, urticaria, eczema), the respiratory system (e.g. hayfever, rhinitis, allergic asthma), the digestive system (e.g. diarrhoea, constipation, 'irritable bowel'), or the nervous system (usually as headaches).

There is unquestionably more allergy around nowadays. It has become more commonplace because of the effects of environmental pollution, thereby increasing the allergic 'load' the population has to carry. Some people are able to deal with this, others are less so.

Nevertheless, it should be pointed out that in recent times allergy has become a bit of a 'fad'. It is probable that far too many symptoms are being attributed to allergy, especially food allergy (which should really in most cases be called food intolerance or food sensitivity. A true food allergy is a severe reaction involving very severe symptoms); following testing by often unreliable means many people are avoiding certain foods unnecessarily because they have been told they are 'allergic' to them.

Because of the lack of help by doctors in general practice, many people are also resorting to self-diagnosis and the use of restricted diets on their own account by reading books and literature on the subject, and while many of these efforts are helpful and successful, many others are not.

Allergy is often thought of as being inevitable or even 'genetic', if relatives or parents have suffered from the same problems. A herbalist will think of these factors as lending a *tendency* towards allergy, as the bodily organs in a family line tend to work in a similar pattern of imbalance (or of good balance). However, a pattern of imbalance does not mean an inevitable outcome, since if the organs can be helped to work differently, then the pattern can change in the case of any individual.

This point is demonstrated by the fact that frequently some members of a family, *but not all*, have similar allergies; if allergies were inevitable then *all* the family members would be condemned to the same degree of allergy, since all have inherited the same genetic pattern. The difference is accounted for by the variable functioning of the organs responsible for allergy in these different family members.

In treating allergies or intolerances, a herbalist will once again follow the example of nature itself as the model for treatment. We can clearly see that the body is able to heal itself of allergies, as evidenced by the fact that you will often hear people say that they *used to have* this or that allergy (for instance hayfever), but now they do not. Or, conversely, that they *never used to have* this or that allergy, but now they do.

The proper conclusion from this is that allergy is not a fixed state, or an inevitability, but a fluid one that the body can move into or out of. The intention behind herbal treatment, therefore, is to encourage the body to heal itself from an allergy or intolerance, in the same way that it is clearly capable of doing on its own, in certain circumstances.

The beginning of this natural treatment of allergies is in understanding the fact that allergies occur *within the body of the sufferer*: it is so easy to *externalize* allergies, to see them as something that is being done *to* the body of the sufferer, and not *by* their body.

This is clearly shown by the ability of the body to heal itself, often on a cycle of seven years at age seven, fourteen, twenty-one, twenty-eight, etc. When an allergy clears up in this way, the same substance, which has not in itself changed, no longer produces the same allergic reaction within the sufferer, thus indicating clearly that the allergy was in the sufferer, not within the substance.

Additional evidence to support this is provided by the fact that not everyone reacts in an allergic way to pollen, for instance. If there were something inevitably allergenic (allergy-producing) about pollen, then everyone would react in the same way to pollen; since they clearly do not, then the allergy must be within the sufferer and not carried by the allergenic substance itself.

So allergy is a representation of the state of reactivity of the body of the sufferer to foreign substances. The degree of reactivity is excessive, there is increased bodily activity and an exaggerated immune response which provokes inflammation in particular areas of the body in different people (e.g. the nasal passages, the eyes, the face, the lips, the skin in general, the lungs, the bowels, the nervous system), and this inflammation triggers off the symptoms which are noticed, such as weeping eyes, a runny nose, wheezing, diarrhoea, as the body comes under the effect of the resultant overactivity and tries to clear itself of the excess heat or inflammation.

Therefore allergy may be viewed as something which can point out to us that there is hyper-reactivity in the body, and not necessarily as something which 'should not be happening' or which has no value. If we learn from allergy to regain and to seek better health, and to make changes that are necessary, then it will have served its purpose.

Most herbalists would agree that there is a place for anti-histamines or adrenaline as treatments for severe and emergency cases of allergy, but would also contend that beyond such emergency treatments the deeper imbalances in the functioning of the immune system, the adrenal glands and the digestive system in particular, as the organs responsible both for producing and for reducing allergic reactions, should be addressed.

In their customary way, herbalists treat the whole of the person with attention to all the organs involved in allergy; they include in their treatment dietary changes appropriate to the individual, such as the avoidance of cow's milk or wheat, or a yeast-reduction regime, and take into account stress (which many allergy sufferers will confirm often makes their allergic reactions worse) in their selection of herbs for any one individual.

6   RHEUMATISM AND ARTHRITIS

ORTHODOX DRUG TREAMENT   People with arthritis or rheumatism are often told by their doctor that it is virtually an inevitability as one gets older, that there is nothing that can be done about it as there is no identifiable cause, it is just something that happens, that it will almost certainly get worse, and that the only treatment is a palliative one by taking anti-inflammatory drugs, painkillers (some of which can be addictive), and steroids at a later stage if the disease progresses and they become necessary. This may be followed by bone replacement operations in certain suitable cases once the disease has reached an advanced stage. It is rare for doctors to give advice about diet or to suggest that the patient may gain some help by eliminating certain foods.

HERBAL TREATMENT   Fortunately, this gloomy picture painted by orthodox medicine is not accepted by everyone, and some people take matters into their own hands and start experimenting with their diet, leaving out certain foods or changing the combination of foods they eat together, or investigating the issue of food intolerance for themselves, often after having come across some media account of someone who has got better by this means.

For such people herbal medicine can be helpful, since herbalists see arthritis and rheumatism as the end result of a chronic (meaning long-term) degeneration that has been taking place in the joints of the body, usually for many years before it shows up as the stiffness and pain that are generally the first symptoms that the sufferer feels.

The reason that a change in diet is usually necessary is that certain foods in certain people can cause the *inflammation* that underlies the whole problem, and that leads to the swelling and pain that result. So it is necessary to recommend that these foods be removed from the sufferer's diet to allow a reduction in this heat or inflammation throughout the system. Whilst generalization is not possible, foods containing a high level of acidity are often found to be unhelpful in arthritis, since acid is heat-producing.

The herbs that are used in arthritis and rheumatism are aimed at improving elimination of this heat and toxicity from the system, herbs with a diuretic (fluid-removing), or laxative, or diaphoretic (sweat-inducing) action, as may be appropriate to the individual case.

Whilst no cure can be promised by a herbalist in any one particular case, often in practice it *is* possible, with the right advice on diet and the right herbs for the particular person, to at least arrest or stop the progression of the disease, and this in itself is a worthwhile achievement for many sufferers of these degenerative conditions.

8
•••••

Side-effects and Safety

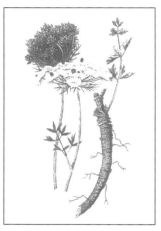

CARROT
Daucus carota

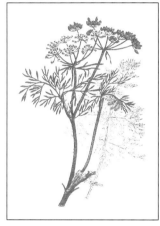

CARAWAY
Carum carvi

H erbalists are often asked by patients whether herbs have any 'side-effects'. Side-effect means an effect not intended by the treatment itself, often on another part of the body, for instance the contraceptive Pill and hormone replacement therapy (HRT) often raise the blood pressure, which is a side-effect.

Side-effects from drug medicines are common enough and are so accepted and acknowledged, that there is a whole reporting system for them by doctors. The reason for drug side-effects is that since the body is an integrated whole, it is not possible for one part of it to be affected by a treatment without all other parts also being affected. Thus, a drug having a therapeutic effect in one part of the body will inevitably have an effect elsewhere. This effect may be very minimal, but it may also be quite major, for example, aspirin may cause liver damage. Because it is such a common expression in medical circles, people are now quite understandably asking whether herbs, too, can have side-effects.

In regard to herbal medicines, it is actually inaccurate to say that they can have *side-effects*: they may have *toxic* effects if poisonous herbs are taken, or they may have *adverse* effects if inappropriate herbs are taken, but these are not the same as side-effects, which refer only to the actions of drug medicines.

As an example, St John's Wort is sometimes referred to as having a side-effect of photosensitivity (increased sensitivity to light) in some people. This is, in fact, an inaccuracy, since this reaction does not occur in people who are suited to this herb, only in people who are not suited to it, by paradoxically increasing their nervous system activity to the point where photosensitivity occurs. Thus, photosensitivity caused by St John's Wort is an *adverse* effect and not a side-effect, experienced by people whom it does not suit. This is bound to occur where large numbers of people are taking it without any professional advice.

Closely connected to this issue is another question that herbalists are frequently asked: 'Are herbal medicines safe?'

The answer has to be: 'Not necessarily'.

There are, in fact, two aspects to this matter. Firstly, herbs may be taken by a person without full knowledge of their actions in the human body, leading to a physiological change in their body that is *inappropriate*. An example of this would be someone taking certain types of Ginseng for 'stress' or 'more energy' who has high blood pressure already. Since it is a fact that *some* types of Ginseng can actually raise the blood pressure, it would obviously be inappropriate and inadvisable for them to take it in this case.

This is an example not of a herb being dangerous in itself, since many people take Ginseng to great benefit, but rather of the *use* of it being ill-advised and inappropriate to the person in question.

Secondly, there is the question of the constituent parts of herbs possibly being poisonous or toxic. There is no doubt that herbs do contain many substances which *in isolation* (in other words, taken by chemical extraction out of their naturally-occurring context or state in a laboratory) would be toxic to the human system.

Herbalists have to be aware which herbal medicines they use could have an action of possible toxicity, and use these medicines in *limited dose*. Some of these medicines are only available through a herbalist, after a consultation with the individual patient, which is another argument in favour of the profession of herbalist or herbal practitioner being an officially-recognized one, so that the public may be re-assured that they are taking advice from a professional practitioner who is aware of the possible dangers of herbal medicines.

In a more general sense we should not think that because plants contain chemical components which in isolation might be toxic, this makes the plant toxic as a medicine. The balance of *all* the components in the plant as a whole seems to regulate any toxic effect of individual components, in plants that are traditionally used as medicines. This is known as *synergy*, where the effect of the whole is different to the sum of the effects of all the different parts, and is another example of the *balance* bestowed by nature.

Never forget, though, that some plants *are poisonous*.

Standardized Extracts of Herbal Medicines

Certain manufacturers claim that the herbal medicines which they have chemically altered in the laboratory contain more of what they call the active components than Nature intended and are therefore superior to the plant in its natural state.

A true herbalist would not hold to this view at all. Nature has provided the plant as a medicine for mankind in its natural state: there may be variations in the chemical components from plant to plant and from one batch of herbal medicine to the next batch, but the overall balance of the constituents is as nature intended.

It is an arrogant stance by an over-scientific mind to suggest that man can improve on nature, when man's knowledge is so incomplete in any case. It may be that a component in the medicine whose proportion to the whole is reduced by such 'pharmaceuticalization' of herbs is the very one that will later be discovered to be vital to the overall effect. So herbalists would fundamentally disagree with the chemical alteration of plants for medicines, and only use herbs in their complete, unaltered, and natural state.

The recent controversy over St John's Wort was based mainly on apparent evidence including just such chemically-altered versions of the plant. It must be obvious to anyone that if you alter a natural substance you are going to get different effects than if you use it in its naturally-occurring form. For the same reason herbalists would not agree with the use of genetically-modified plants for herbal medicines, since there is no reason to suppose that they will have the same properties as plants that occur naturally, which do have medicinal properties. Man plays with Nature at his peril.

9

• • • • •

Five Case Histories

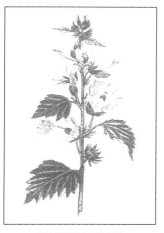

MARSH MALLOW
Althæa officinalis

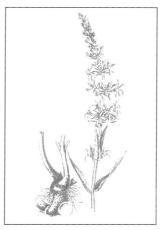

PURPLE LOOSESTRIFE
Lythrum salicaria

T he following case histories have been chosen to illustrate the key principles of herbal medicine as discussed in this guide. The choice was made also with a view to showing a range of conditions that a herbalist treats, including those that have been successful as well as those where there were variations in success – typical of herbal practice.

It is hoped that these case notes will be of interest and understandable to both the general public and to orthodox doctors, especially those who are interested in understanding more about the practice of herbal medicine.

CASE 1: IBS

FIRST VISIT

F emale patient aged 70, first presented with 'irritable bowel syndrome' (IBS), (doctor's diagnosis). Onset several years previously, worsened two months before first visit following mild gastric infection. Had seen doctor many times over the years, no help with condition, no dietary advice by doctor. Had two years previously had allergy testing on own initiative privately – cow's milk intolerance indicated: had helped with condition. Problem now constant since re-occurrence. Main symptoms complained of: bowel urgency, 3–4 motions per day, liquid and yellow stools. Bowel may also not move for up to 3 days.

Other symptoms found on questioning: stress/frustration due to domestic tension; hot sweats during the night (doctor tells her to keep using HRT despite no improvement).

Relevant past medical history: salmonella-poisoning approx. 8 years previously.

Drugs taken: hormone replacement therapy patch (HRT) for 4 years, Loperamide hydrochloride (anti-diarrhoeal), Propranolol hydrochloride (beta-blocker to reduce blood pressure) for approx. 5 years.

Relevant drug side-effects:

HRT: liver function possibly affected leading to variable bowel habit; patient's appearance also yellow indicative of liver being affected.

Loperamide: constipation ? (patient occasionally going up to 3 days with no bowel motion).

Propranolol: gastro-intestinal disturbances possible.

Diet: General diet with low vegetable and fibre intake (adverse effect on bowel, worsening the diarrhoea). Following allergy testing – no milk (using soya milk), but not avoiding all products of cow's milk: still having cheese and butter.

ASSESSMENT AND DIAGNOSIS:
Multi-factorial picture with probable salmonella infection-induced origin, cow's milk intolerance but not doing complete cow's milk restriction diet, probable unhelpful drug side-effects, and stress factor tending to induce nervous diarrhoea.

STRATEGY:
Gave diet sheet for complete avoidance of all cow's milk products.

Suggested cessation of Loperamide and HRT patch.

Reduce emotional stress and bowel tension using relaxant herbs. Had conversation about domestic stress to try to facilitate solution.

Reduce loose motions and improve liver function using astringent herbs beneficial to the liver.

HERBAL PRESCRIPTION:
Combined tincture of (millilitres/mls. per week) –
Berberis aquifolium (Mountain grape)	10
Mentha piperita (Peppermint)	10
Chamomilla recutita (Chamomile)	30
Potentilla erecta (Tormentil)	30
Agrimonia eupatoria (Agrimony)	10
Chondrus crispus (Irish Moss)	40
Scutellaria laterifolia (Skullcap)	20

Sig. 10 ml. bd. aq. gel. a.c.
(10 ml. taken twice daily in cold water before food).

☐

SECOND VISIT

Two weeks later.

Had followed dairy-free diet.

Had stopped HRT patch and Loperamide. Had seen doctor and changed from Propranolol to Felodipine (no side-effects on bowel) for blood pressure: to be monitored by doctor now on new drug.

CONDITION:
No bowel urgency, no yellow stools, diarrhoea very much reduced. Only once had more than one motion per day. Had 3 or 4 days without a bowel motion, but only for 1 day.

Stress said to be lessened, feels calmer about domestic situation.

Still suffering hot spells in night.

STRATEGY:
Get bowel moving every day by increasing liver enzyme production.

Address hormone imbalance leading to hot spells at night by restoring function of adrenal glands and reducing body heat in general.

HERBAL PRESCRIPTION:

Combined tincture of (millilitres/mls. per week)	–
Berberis aquifolium	10
Mentha piperita	10
Chondrus crispus	30
Scutellaria laterifolia	30
Hypericum perforatum (St John's Wort)	30
Borago officinalis (Borage)	34
Chelidonium majus (Greater Celandine)	6
(Taken as before)	

☐

THIRD VISIT

Six weeks later.

CONDITION:
No bowel symptoms at all for past four weeks, except 4 days prior to visit when got 'worked up' about having blood pressure monitored at doctor's. Going once daily, no urgency, no missed days.

No hot spells at night for past five weeks or so.

Still pursuing dairy-free diet.

Only drug now the new one for blood pressure.

HERBAL PRESCRIPTION:
Combined tincture of (millilitres/mls. per week)	–
Berberis aq.	10
Mentha pip.	10
Hypericum perf.	40
Scutellaria lat.	40
Borago off.	34
Chelidonium majus	6
(Taken as before).	

SIX WEEKS LATER

Condition very satisfactory.

Repeat prescription without consultation at half dose for further 4 weeks, then treatment ends.

CASE 2: FACIAL ACNE

FIRST VISIT

F emale patient aged 21, presenting with facial acne: considerable erythema (redness), and spots with yellow pus; all of face affected, worsening at time of attendance in both severity and rate of outbreak. Onset aged 15–16. Not said to be connected to menstrual (period) cycle. Had tried many different creams, and herbal and homeopathic remedies bought herself. Had been prescribed two six-month courses of tetracycline antibiotics, and most recently an oral contraceptive given for acne, Cyproterone acetate with ethinyloestradiol: she had stopped this four weeks before her first visit having taken it for 18 months, as it had not been effective enough and had worsened the frequency of headaches.

Other symptoms on questioning: menstrual cycle of habitually 24–5 days when not on contraceptive Pill. (This is too short and indicative of a hormone imbalance.) Tender breasts and other fluid retention pre-menstrually. Three severe attacks of 'hives' in past 2 years (all-over, red, hot rash with itching). Had been diagnosed by doctor as having a fungal chest infection 2 years ago. Bowels not moving daily, 5–6 days per week only (long-standing pattern). Cheese produces feeling of nausea. Throbbing headaches, made worse by movement, and tendency to feel over-hot, especially during a headache. Some factor of overwork, and resultant stress (anxiety) and tiredness, in connection with headaches.

Drugs taken: painkillers as required for headaches.

Diet: Low-fat diet, which had been of some help to her skin. Diet rather low in salads and vegetables.

ASSESSMENT AND DIAGNOSIS:
Deduced a yeast-intolerance from symptoms of previous fungal chest infection and attacks of hives. Antibiotics for acne would have been unhelpful to yeast-intolerance by lowering immune system function. Insufficient elimination of metabolic residues of yeast excess and hormone-derived toxicity, as well as general systemic inflammation/heat build-up, due to poor liver function and consequent deficient bowel function, leading to skin becoming a means of elimination (=acne).

STRATEGY:
- Yeast-free diet sheet given to lower systemic yeast level.
- No coffee (mildly hepatotoxic - unhelpful to liver function).
- Increase in salads and vegetables suggested, and also in water intake.
- Herbs to improve bowel function to daily evacuation, reduce systemic inflammation, improve elimination of toxins through kidneys also, redress hormone imbalance reflecting in short monthly menstrual cycle, and improve resistance to mild systemic fungal excess.

HERBAL PRESCRIPTION:
Combined tincture of (millilitres/mls. per week)	–
Chelidonium majus (Greater Celandine)	5
Berberis aquifolium (Mountain Grape)	10

Chamomilla recutita (Chamomile)	15
Urtica dioica (Nettle)	25
Fucus vesiculosus (Kelp)	25
Alchemilla vulgaris (Lady's Mantle)	20
Valeriana officinalis (Valerian)	20
Echinacea angustifolia (Echinacea)	20

Sig. 10 ml. sd aq. gel. p.c.
(10 ml. taken once daily in cold water after food).

☐

SECOND VISIT

Four weeks later.

Had followed yeast-reduction diet with only occasional lapse. Had increased vegetable intake, and avoided coffee.

CONDITION:
Acne considerably improved, hardly any yellow pus in spots and a slowdown in production of spots. One mild bout of hives. Bowel moving daily now, sometimes twice daily. Only two headaches. No change in period cycle or in pre-menstrual fluid retention.

STRATEGY:
Continue process of toxin elimination and reduction of consequent inflammation, via bowel and kidneys; increase gentle stimulation of correct balance of hormones with reference to length of period cycle (28–29 days being normal).

HERBAL PRESCRIPTION:

Combined tincture of (millilitres/mls. per week)	–
Chelidonium majus	5
Berberis aquifolium	5
Chamomilla recutita	25
Urtica dioica	20
Fucus vesiculosus	25
Alchemilla vulgaris	25
Valeriana officinalis	20
Echinacea angustifolia	20

Vitex agnus-castus (Chasteberry)   5
(Taken as before)

☐

THIRD VISIT

Ten weeks later.

CONDITION:
Continued gradual improvement in acne, hardly any new spots emerging now; only very small amount of yellow pus occasionally. One more bout of hives (mild). Bowel continuing to move at least once daily. Only two headaches in ten weeks (very good improvement), lasting a few hours only, not lingering, no need for painkillers; still hot during a headache. Period cycle: first period after last visit was a 30-day cycle, second one was 28 days (which is normal, indicating correct balance in hormones); there had been no fluid retention or breast tenderness before either of these two periods.

STRATEGY:
Continue improvement of functioning of organs of elimination (of toxicity); adjustment of prescription to include different herbs helpful to liver; continue to address excessive heat in body by addition of further herbs beneficial to function of adrenal glands.

HERBAL PRESCRIPTION:
Combined tincture of (millilitres/mls. per week)   –

Chelidonium majus	2.5
Berberis aquifolium	2.5
Chamomilla recutita	20
Urtica dioica	15
Fucus vesiculosus	20
Alchemilla vulgaris	25
Valeriana officinalis	10
Echinacea angustifolia	15
Vitex agnus-castus	5
Scutellaria laterifolia (Skullcap)	15
Taraxacum officinalis (radix) (Dandelion Root)	2.5
Arctium lappa (Burdock)	2.5

| Borago officinalis (Borage) | 12.5 |
| Trifolium pratense (Red Clover) | 2.5 |

(Taken as before)

Patient still under treatment at time of writing.

CASE 3: 'ACID STOMACH'

FIRST VISIT

F emale aged 69 complaining of 'acid stomach' with onset 3 weeks previously, following a severely stressful situation regarding her work, the particular event being described by her as 'like a bereavement', and which had been going on for a number of months. Attacks of acidity last 3–4 hours, with severe central chest pain, a choking sensation, and nausea.

She had previously had the same condition 2 years ago, and had been prescribed and taken the drug Ranitidine (an ulcer-healing drug) for approximately 1 year.

As well as Ranitidine three weeks ago, the doctor had prescribed both Atenolol (a Beta-blocker used in angina and high blood pressure) and Bendrofluazide (a diuretic used for high blood pressure) for the past two weeks; her blood pressure, apparently usually 160/60 for years, had gone higher (180/80) three months before the onset of the presenting complaint, at around the time that the stressful events had occurred.

This was known because her blood pressure was under regular monitoring, as she had been taking Thyroxine (artificial thyroid hormone) since 1993, having previously had treatment by both drugs (for a number of years) and then by radioactive iodine (1993) for an *overactive* thyroid gland. (The radioactive treatment had induced a lack of thyroid hormone thus necessitating Thyroxine.)

The dose of Thyroxine had been changed from time to time according to her regular tests for thyroxine level, and on a more loose arrangement according to how she felt (under her doctor's supervision).

She reported that one or other of the two most recently prescribed drugs was making her experience nausea, anorexia (loss of appetite), and 'turning her legs to jelly'.

She was using Hawthorn and Dandelion leaf herbal teas (taken on own initiative), and an over-the-counter multimineral supplement.

Her blood pressure on this first visit was 165/80. On further questioning: recent cholesterol level on blood test of 8.0 but no dietary advice given by doctor.

Drugs being taken: Thyroxine 125/150 mcg. daily, Ranitidine, Bendrofluazide, Atenolol.

Diet: Good quality foods, high intake of vegetables, fruit and salads, but with very high intake of butter. No coffee taken now, as found to irritate her digestive system. No spicy foods for same reason.

ASSESSMENT AND DIAGNOSIS:
Over-acidity in stomach/duodenum, appearing to be precipitated by nervous system overactivity due to stressful events over past few months. Previous history of same problem would appear to confirm diagnosis of gastric inflammation. Blood pressure also probably related to stress, but could also or in part be a side-effect of Thyroxine dose being ? too high.

STRATEGY:
Patient already had appointment with doctor for following week for a 'sort out'.

Also had appointment set up by doctor for six weeks' time with a Cardiologist (heart Consultant).

- Gave dietary suggestions: reduction of butter, no red meats at all, increased use of olive oil.

- Reduce emotional stress using relaxant herbs, which should also help blood pressure (if raised blood pressure not because Thyroxine dose too high).

- Use herbs also to reduce stomach acidity.

HERBAL PRESCRIPTION:

Combined herbal tea of mixed   –

Chamomile flowers	50 (gms.)
Meadowsweet	25
Yarrow	25
Skullcap	50
Motherwort	25

Four cups to be taken daily, using two teaspoons per cup.
The herbal medicine to be commenced after she had seen her doctor
for a review.

SECOND VISIT

Three weeks later.

Had followed dietary advice precisely.

Had commenced the herbal medicine after seeing her doctor,
therefore had been taking the herbs for two weeks: after
commencing the herbal medicine she had not used Ranitidine
or Atenolol, but continued to use Bendrofluazide at the doctor's
request. There had been no need to use the higher (150 mcg.)
dose of Thyroxine at all. She had expressed dissatisfaction to
her doctor that he had put her on medication for angina
without justification, and the improvement she had now
experienced showed it was not angina, as also did the same
experience of two years previously. Her blood pressure at the
doctor's appointment was 160/90.

CONDITION:
The acidity problem was almost completely better, with barely
any symptoms at all for the past week. Feeling well in herself,
much less worried and stressed, much more relaxed, more
energy.

Blood pressure at this visit 180/80.

STRATEGY:
She intended to stop Bendrofluazide after the current
prescription ended, as she did not want to take unnecessary
drugs.

To have blood pressure monitored 4-weekly by nurse at doctor's clinic.

Continue to treat nervous system overactivity with relaxant herbs, and anti-acid herbs for stomach disorder.

HERBAL PRESCRIPTION:

Combined herbal tea of mixed	—
Chamomile flowers	50 (gms.)
Meadowsweet	50
Yarrow	25
Skullcap	50
Motherwort	25
(Taken as before).	

THIRD VISIT

Fourteen weeks later.

CONDITION:
No digestive problems whatsoever.

Had stopped Bendrofluazide soon after last visit. Thyroxine dose now 125 or 150 mcg. again as appropriate.

Blood pressure 180/80 (monitoring by nurse said to be lower than this figure, and doctor satisfied with blood pressure).

STRATEGY:
Continue with herbal tea while she finds it necessary.

Has cholesterol re-check coming up.

CASE 4: ME

FIRST VISIT

M ale aged 53, presented with ME (myalgic encephalo-myelitis). Onset 7 years previously, following severe repetitious flu virus with chest infection. Symptoms: severe and permanent exhaustion, continual (daily) headaches, severely aching joints throughout body, continual sharp stabbing pains in muscles, inflamed and swollen glands, general hotness and spells of excessive sweating. Static condition with heavy drug regime (see below). No spells of remission (improvement).

Other symptoms found on questioning and examination: some chest pain on occasions; loose bowel motions with excessive flatulence; feeling worse approx. 30–60 mins. after food; anxiety over minor events nowadays; apparent ringworm (fungal) infection on chest, chronic (long-standing) condition; recent need for anti-fungal cream for fungal groin infection; blood pressure 170/120, pulse overstrong with some irregularity in rhythm.

Relevant past medical history: ex-serviceman, with many vaccinations and inoculations for tropical travel in past; several repeated courses of antibiotics in 1960s for infected cyst in leg; polio aged 1; chickenpox aged 35.

Drugs taken at first visit: Fluoxetine (antidepressant) for past 6 years for ME. Trimipramine (antidepressant) as sleeping agent for past 5 years. Opiate analgesics (addictive) of two different types, daily over past 6 years for muscle and joint pains.

Aspirin (self-medicated) for past 20 years or so (due to his apparently unfounded concern that he might have a stroke).

Other product taken: over-the-counter 'antioxidant' tablet recently started.

Relevant drug side-effects:
Fluoxetine: sweating, adverse effect on liver.
Trimipramine: sedation, arrythmia (irregular heart rhythm), sweating, adverse effect on liver and immune system.
Opiates: drowsiness, sweating, mood changes.
Aspirin: adverse effect on liver and immune system possible in long-term use.

Diet: good standard of diet with low intake of sugar (sugar affects his symptoms adversely); quite heavy reliance on yeast-based spreads, and on tea; no alcohol as makes feel ill.

ASSESSMENT AND DIAGNOSIS:

Fundamentally, liver severely affected (possibly by heavy receipt of multiple vaccinations in past), leading to low immune system function and consequent permanent aching flu-like symptoms. Chickenpox aged 35 and repeated fungal infections are also symptoms of low immune function, as well as the permanently swollen glands. 'Post-viral fatigue syndrome' would also be a relevant name for this person's condition. Current heavy administration of drugs, both prescribed and self-medicated, almost certainly unhelpful due mainly to their inhibiting effects on liver function and immune system.

STRATEGY:

- Need to reduce yeast (fungal) level, so yeast-reduction diet given.
- Gradual reduction of Opiate (addictive drug) and Trimipramine, over 4-week period to ensure safe withdrawal (gave reduction chart to guide withdrawal).
- Recommended cessation of Aspirin, as apparently unwarranted: suggested blood test to check on blood quality after a few weeks without it.
- Herbal medicine to improve liver function and immunity, and to relax whole of nervous system, and thus help muscular aches and high blood pressure probably caused in part by muscular tension as well as exhaustion.

HERBAL PRESCRIPTION:

Combined tincture of (millilitres/mls. per week)   –

Echinacea angustifolia (Echinacea)	70
Hypericum perforatum (St John's Wort)	70
Scutellaria laterifolia (Skullcap)	70

Sig. 10 ml. tds. aq.gel.

(10 mls. to be taken in cold water three times daily, having soaked the tincture overnight in water to de-alcoholise it).

SECOND VISIT

Two weeks later.

Had followed dietary advice completely.

Had halved dose of both Trimipramine and Opiate, and stopped Aspirin.

Still taking Fluoxetine.

CONDITION:
Still extremely tired as before, but with the beginnings of some feeling of well-being on occasions now. Headaches no longer continuous, some clear spells of a few hours now. Glands less tender, and gone down in size on right-hand side. Sharp muscular pains and general joint aches unchanged. Sweating considerably decreased but still present.

Blood pressure 165/105, pulse still overstrong but now regular.

STRATEGY:
Continue same objectives.

HERBAL PRESCRIPTION:
Combined tincture of (millilitres/mls. per week)	—
Echinacea angustifolia	60
Hypericum perforatum	75
Scutellaria laterifolia	75
(Taken as before).	

THIRD VISIT

Three weeks later.

Continued dietary restrictions as before.

Now completely off Trimipramine , and only taking occasional Opiate for neck and shoulder pain.

Fluoxetine as before.

Now taking Paracetamol for pain on 3-4 days a week.

CONDITION:
General lift of energy, able to go for a walk now. Headaches only in afternoons. Glands less swollen and tender to touch. Muscle aches and joint pains had improved but now returning again. Better quality of sleep, but broken pattern. Mood: now feeling 'hopeful' for first time for years. Blood pressure 150/105.

STRATEGY:
Continue muscular relaxation and beneficial effect of herbs on
liver. Encourage gentle metabolic rate normalization using Kelp
(a seaweed). Reduce Fluoxetine by 1/4 dose weekly over 4 weeks.

HERBAL PRESCRIPTION:
Combined tincture of (millilitres/mls. per week)   –
(i)
Scutellaria laterifolia   75
Viburnum opulus (Guelder Rose)   75
Sig 10 ml. bd.
(10 ml. taken twice daily)

(ii)
Kelp 200 mg. tablets.
Sig. 3 tablets bd.
(3 tablets twice daily).

FOURTH VISIT

Four weeks later.

No drug medication at all now.

Continued diet as before.

CONDITION:
Considerable relapse on reduction of Fluoxetine dose. All
symptoms returned almost to original state. Also reported
tingling in hands and feet. Sleep the worst problem now;
palpitations (feeling the heart beat) on lying down to sleep.
Blood pressure 150/105.

Pulse regular, overstrong still.

Another factor emerged more clearly on discussion: patient
beset during night by images of combat experienced in services,
very distressing experiences.

STRATEGY:
• Resume Fluoxetine for 3 months to allow body to further
  adjust to withdrawal of other drugs, and having to work on
  its own now without drug interference. (Possibly Fluoxetine
  could remain as a continued treatment if necessary,
  depending on how progress goes.)

- Suggested hypnotherapy for traumatic events experienced: patient willing to consider this.

- Suggested reduction of high tea intake, or decaffeinated tea instead, as blood pressure not coming down low enough. Herbs to support nervous system and liver further, and now also herbs to benefit heart and adrenal glands function.

HERBAL PRESCRIPTION:

Combined tincture of (millilitres/mls. per week)   –
(i)

Hypericum perforatum	50
Echinacea angustifolia	10
Crategus oxycanthoides (Hawthorn berries)	50
Borago officinalis (Borage)	50

(Taken as before)

(ii)
Kelp tablets (taken as before).

FIFTH VISIT

Three weeks later.

Now on Fluoxetine only.

Had avoided tea.

CONDITION:
All symptoms still present to some degree, but now very much less severe than ever before. Glands now normal.

Had seen hypnotherapist and treatment successful, no longer kept awake by unpleasant images, and therefore sleeping wonderfully at night.

Reported feeling of growing well-being, and said he now believes he can get better for the first time.

Blood pressure 150/100.

STRATEGY:
Continue same objectives. Addition of herbal tea to increase beneficial effect on liver and nervous system.

HERBAL PRESCRIPTION:

Combined tincture of (millilitres/mls. per week)   –

(i)

Hypericum perforatum	60
Echinacea angustifolia	20
Crategus oxycanthoides	60
Borago officinalis	60
Gentiana lutea (Gentian)	10

Sig. 30 ml. sd.

(30 ml. to be taken once daily)

(ii)

Continue Kelp tablets.

(iii)

Vervain herb (as tea).

Take 3 cups daily using 1 teaspoon per cup.

Patient remains on herbal treatment 8 months later, now stopped Fluoxetine without ill-effect. Also, now able to walk freely and almost pain-free.

CASE 5: INFANT ECZEMA

FIRST VISIT

M ale child aged 15 months, presented with eczema. Onset aged 3 months. Very dry skin inflammation covering neck, arms, wrists, ankles. Treatments tried: various moisturising creams from doctor, for past 6 months steroid (hydrocortisone) creams of increasing strength from own doctor and then Dermatologist; Marigold (herbal) cream (bought by mother over-the-counter); had seen a homeopath for treatment of 3 months' duration in past. 3 courses of antibiotics necessary in past 12 months for skin infections related to eczema. Over-the-counter Echinacea (herbal) drops seem to have helped in past.

Pursuing cow's milk-free diet for past 4 weeks at first visit (not really effecting any benefit).

Other symptoms on questioning: very hot person (especially at night), with frequent heat-rashes. Very active, almost hyperactive, with boundless, excessive energy too late into the evenings for his age. Clammyness (dampness) present by way of tendency to sweat profusely, again especially at night. Other physiological processes normal otherwise, except some incidence of chest infections with 2 courses of antibiotics necessary in history.

Drugs taken: steroid (hydrocortisone) cream as required (not daily due to parents' reluctance to use it more than absolutely necessary).

Diet:

Excellent quality general diet due to parents' considerable dietary awareness and efforts to not eat 'junk' foods. Currently on cow's milk-free diet.

Assessment and diagnosis:

Person with overactive physiology leading to excessive generation of heat and resultant eczema (as body endeavours to rid itself of the excess heat), as well as a tendency to hyperactivity (goes with body heat). Slightly lowered immunity leading to chest infections and infected skin at times.

STRATEGY:
• Abandon cow's milk-free diet, as no help.
• Reduce limited amount of refined sugars and white flour taken, as they generate heat.
• Not to use steroid cream: warned that condition may worsen as steroid cream is withdrawn altogether.
• Aim is to reduce systemic body heat by using anti-inflammatory herbs to reduce actual (blood-borne) inflammation, and to increase adrenal glands' capacity to deal with inflammation: this should result in a calmer, cooler child whose body has no need to manifest eczema as there would then be no excessive body heat.

HERBAL PRESCRIPTION:

Combined tincture of (millilitres/mls. per week)   –

(i) Combined tincture of (millilitres/mls. per week):

Urtica dioica (Nettle)	10
Borago officinalis (Borage)	12.5
Scutellaria laterifolia (Skullcap)	5
Verbascum thapsus (Mullein)	5
Berberis aquifolium (Mountain Grape)	2.5

Sig. 100 gtt. sd.

(100 drops/5 mls. to be taken daily).

(ii) Marigold and Chickweed (combined) herbal cream.

SECOND VISIT

4 weeks later.

Had followed dietary advice given and also resumed dairy (cow's milk) foods.

No steroid cream used.

CONDITION:

No change in condition of skin, or in general body heat and tendency to hyperactivity.

Discovered that only one half of the herbal medicine had been taken. Herbal cream had been used.

STRATEGY:

Continue with diet and take herbal medicine at correct dose.

Repeat herbal prescription to allow for four weeks. Repeat herbal cream.

THIRD VISIT

4 weeks later.

Had continued dietary advice given.

No steroid cream used or necessary.

CONDITION:
Eczema almost gone by end of first two weeks of treatment.

Herbal medicine had been stopped by parents one week before second visit, as eczema had all but disappeared! Worsening of eczema had begun again after three days or so of stopping medicine.

Much calmer generally, and considerably less hot and sweaty at night.

STRATEGY:
• Continue excellent progress.

HERBAL PRESCRIPTION:
Finish remaining medicine and repeat tincture as before.

FOURTH VISIT

Six weeks later.

CONDITION:
No eczema for three weeks. Medicine and cream almost finished.

STRATEGY:
Discharged. Return in future if necessary.

10
•••••

Current Position in Orthodox Western Medical Healthcare

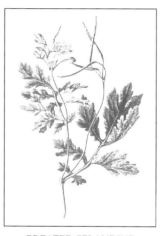

GREATER CELANDINE
Chelidonium majus

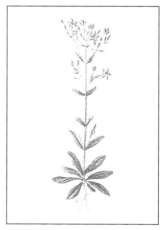

CENTAURY
Erythræa centaurium

W hen a person is unwell, she or he will most often first visit a qualified doctor or registered medical practitioner. In the English-speaking world this means consulting a person trained primarily, and usually only, in the use of chemical drugs as a means of treating illnesses.

There are very few doctors with little more than a cursory or very sketchy knowledge of other forms of treatment. Some will have done short courses in alternative or complementary medicine – usually over a three or four-week period. This hardly compares with a professional training in herbal medicine, which takes place over four or five years, and involves real experience in the traditional use of herbal medicine as a therapy in its own right.

The fundamental difference between herbal medicine and chemical medicine is that chemical medicines intervene in the physiological processes of the body by artificially inducing an action into the living system: this runs *against* what the person's own body is trying to do (since the body only ever does what it needs to do), and is therefore termed *allopathic*, meaning an alien or foreign action within the body.

Immediately, therefore, we can see a problem: the person who may favour natural forms of treatment is confronted in their doctor with someone whose medical knowledge, in most cases, is limited to the application of chemical drugs.

A number of different scenarios now present themselves, and the author draws on real experiences to summarize these for readers as a possible rehearsal for what may happen to them. Take the treatment of eczema as an example:

1. The doctor diagnoses eczema and prescribes a cream.

2. The patient says she would like to get to the *cause* of the eczema, not just use a cream to disguise or mask the *symptoms* of it.

3. The doctor says it is something people have to live with and she may grow out of it, that there is nothing more she can do about it and she should use the cream until then.

4. The patient says she has heard that some people get better from eczema by successfully using herbal medicine.

   a) The doctor says yes, that is a fantastic idea, and recommends a qualified herbalist in the area.

   b) The doctor says he has no objection and as he does not know anything about herbal medicine the patient should consult a qualified herbalist, preferably going to someone who has been recommended by a friend or acquaintance.

   c) The doctor says the patient should go to a health food shop and seek advice over-the-counter.

   d) The doctor says that since there is no proof that herbal medicine works, the patient would be wasting her money on it. He adds that since it has not been researched it should not be regarded as safe; furthermore that the patient should be aware that some herbal medicines are dangerous and 'can damage your liver'. He adds that if herbal medicine had any value he would be using it himself, and that since he isn't, it can't have any value.

   e) The doctor says if the patient does not want his advice and does not want to do what he tells her, then she should not consult him.

   f) The doctor says that if she does go and see a herbalist he will not be prepared to treat her in the future.

These different scenarios are all taken from experience and happen all the time. They could equally apply to dozens of medical conditions other than eczema that a patient might ask about.

We can see, therefore, that there are a great number of possible outcomes when a patient asks their doctor about the use of herbal medicine in treating an illness. The fact remains, however, that most doctors have trained only in the use of chemical drugs and are not really in a position to comment one way or another on the possible validity of herbal medicine as a treatment for any medical condition.

Of course, if the doctor is in favour, then all goes very smoothly, assuming the treatment is successful: everyone ends up happy.

It is when the doctor is against herbal remedies, that problems arise. The patient may decide not to seek herbal treatment at all, not wishing to go against the doctor's wishes for fear of being 'struck off' the doctor's list and being refused future care. It is unfortunate that this situation is found more often than one would like to believe in clinical practice, especially among older people. Sadly, this sometimes condemns the patient to a long period of suffering from what the doctor calls 'something you have to live with', and in some cases even a lifetime of ever-stronger creams or other drugs.

If the patient does go against the doctor's wishes and seeks help with herbal treatment, she or he is often unwilling to tell the doctor this. What should be a cooperative partnership between doctor and patient becomes a secretive endeavour on the part of the patient to get better despite the doctor's wishes.

If the herbal treatment is successful, the doctor may think that the prescribed cream or drug has been successful and therefore never finds out that it was herbal medicine that benefited the patient. Because of these factors, which occur all the time in actual practice, many patients enter into the use of herbal medicine without informing or consulting their doctor at all, which is regrettable, because we are all supposed to be on the same side in providing patient care and successful treatments, whatever type of medicines we may use as practitioners.

11
• • • • •

A Word on Antibiotics

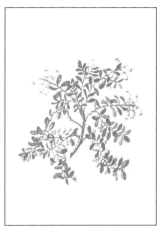

BEARBERRY (UVA-URSI)
Arbutus uva-ursi

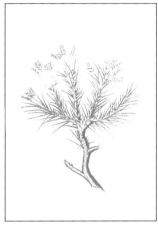

TRAGACANTH
Astragalus gummifer

Drawing on his experience in clinical practice, the author often finds himself saying to his patients that if he could get himself on TV for a two-minute slot just once, he would use it to give one single message to doctors, which would be as follows:

If your patient is allergic to penicillin, what that means is that she or he has too much yeast in her or his gut, and would therefore benefit from a yeast-reduction diet.

The reasons for this being so important in the author's experience are as follows:

1) Doctors do not seem to know what it means when a person is allergic to penicillin, and therefore seem not to be able to give correct advice to patients on health matters which have their origin in this issue.

2) This is a quite common allergy which patients usually know about for themselves because they have had some sort of reaction, often a serious one such as a severe rash, angioedema (swelling), vomiting, or diarrhoea on past exposure to penicillin, and it is generally on their medical record.

3) Penicillin is a strong fungus (yeast is also a fungus), and therefore it is very easy for anyone with common sense and a little depth to their thinking to deduce that *other fungi or yeasts in the diet may also have a similar effect on a patient*.

4) Many foods lead to too much yeast in the human gut or intestine, where a certain level of yeast (*Candida albicans*) already lives as a fungal parasite under normal conditions; when there is too much yeast it can lead to problems, mainly abdominal bloating, flatulence (wind), diarrhoea, constipation (in other words, what is often called by doctors 'irritable bowel

syndrome'), and sudden severe itchy rashes, with or without angioedema (swelling).

5) This is an increasingly common problem, particularly in women, as generations come through who have been brought up on excessive antibiotics and the contraceptive Pill, and now may be using hormone replacement therapy (HRT), all of which can cause thrush (a yeast or fungal infection which indicates too much yeast in the person's system). Much suffering could therefore be easily saved if doctors were aware what it means when a person is allergic to penicillin.

6) Because of the simplicity of this message and the success achieved through explaining this to many hundreds of patients over the past ten years or so, and because of the benefit achieved by patients when they change their diet appropriately, the author believes that if he could be allowed on TV for just a two-minute slot, then probably many more people who have not been helped by their doctors over this issue which is so simple to comprehend, could be saved a great deal of suffering.

The final problem with antibiotics is that, as doctors themselves acknowledge, antibiotics weaken the body's own immune system; they do this by adversely affecting the liver, as it is the liver which has to clear the toxicity caused (antibiotics are very toxic substances). Since the liver is one of the organs where the blood is processed and formed and therefore very central to the immune system, this means that the person often has to be given several courses of antibiotics in succession, because the first course, whilst killing off bacterial infections, in itself makes it more likely that the person will catch another infection, and so a vicious circle of *antibiotic – lowered immunity – infection — antibiotic* is set up which can be difficult to break out of; people are often given two, three or even four courses of antibiotics for such conditions as glue ear (in children), tonsillitis, and cystitis (urinary infection) within a very short period of time such as three to six weeks. The 'record' that the author has come across in his own practice is a child aged 23 months who had been given 24 courses of antibiotics.

The difference and the beauty of herbal medicine for such infections is that herbal medicine improves the body's *own immunity*, so that infections are 'shrugged off' in a normal way, as is the case with any healthy person. After all, we are all exposed to many types of pathogens (infective agents) all the time, the question is whether we go down with the infection or do not go down with it. A healthy immune system is therefore vital to good health, and a weakened immune system is a great handicap to it.

12
• • • • •

Herbal Medicine: A Closer Look [NINE KEY POINTS]

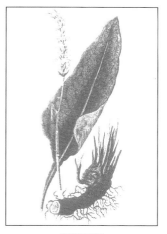

BISTORT
Polygonum bistorta

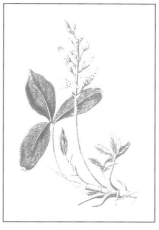

BOGBEAN
Menyanthes trifoliata

'Let your food be your medicine and your medicine be your food'

Hippocrates – the 'Father of Medicine', the most celebrated physician (herbalist) of Greek antiquity (c460–c357BC) and originator of the 'Hippocratic Oath'

T here remain a number of issues about the use of herbal medicine which do not fit neatly into any section so far dealt with, or which need to be revisited. Therefore, this part of the book focuses on a further selection of issues that are often raised in connection with herbal medicine and its place in the modern medical world.

1   A Question of 'Research'

I t is often said by opponents of herbal medicine that, although there may be something in it, 'it hasn't been researched' and is therefore unproven. This is rather like saying that because we do not understand how bees fly, they cannot fly: obviously they *do* fly, and it is our knowledge about how they do it that is deficient, not nature's genius in enabling the bee to fly. Bees do not wait for man to understand how they fly before they do so, they just get on with life; their flight is not dependent on man's approval and understanding.

Herbal medicine is rather like this. Where it works, as thousands of years of mankind's history clearly proves that it often does, it works whether or not we understand how it does so. We do not need to wait until we understand it, it can work for us now as it always has done.

The evidence for the success of herbal medicine may well be what is often disparagingly called an anecdotal one, that is to say people saying that it does, rather than scientists being able to confirm that it does, but what is wrong with anecdotal evidence? We are relying on anecdotal evidence all the time in our normal lives: if a friend says that a restaurant is good, that is anecdotal, and if we go along and also have a good meal we are convinced that their anecdote was correct. Strictly speaking, this may not be scientific proof, but it is what we are all using throughout our lives, and is a part of the human success story.

The other point about the question of research is that both the public and herbalists would welcome it. Research into herbal medicine, however, needs to be undertaken using a radically different format from that in conventional drug medicine, because it is a totally different form of treatment. Research protocols designed for drug medicine will have little value for herbal medicine.

Research needs to include not only the herbal medicines themselves as material entities composed of chemical constituents, but also the role of the herbalist in assessing the patient as a person and a living organism, in directing the whole therapeutic process including the choice of herbs, the dosages, the changing of the prescription, the length of treatment, and many other subtle factors, since as any competent herbalist will tell you these, too, form part of the success of the art of this ancient therapy.

2   The 'Right' Treatment?

I t should not be thought that herbal medicine is the right treatment for every single person: the author's view is that everyone has their right kind of treatment; for many this is drug treatment, where the drug imposes the necessary action which the patient's own body is not doing, and without much need for changes on the part of the patient; this is the right treatment for many people, and therefore they are satisfied with it.

It is when a person begins thinking for themselves about their health, however, that they often see that there is more to good health than merely taking drugs to correct matters on behalf of their own body. Often people then see that 'prevention is better than cure', meaning that if they keep healthy they will not be ill, since these two opposites are incompatible.

Many people, however, *cannot* see that they could not be ill if they were well, and these people are not likely to think about getting their own body working really well for itself, they are content to let their health be a matter that is not especially under their own direction. Such people tend to use orthodox or drug medicine, which will do things for their body rather than think of themselves as responsible for their own health.

More and more younger people, however, are taking their health matters into their own hands. They realize that there is often much that can be done to improve their own and their family's health by natural means, providing that they know what they need to do. This often includes an interest in diet and wholesome food as the first area of interest, and natural treatments such as herbal medicine, aromatherapy, homeopathy and acupuncture.

We find in practice that the best guide to the right treatment for any individual is what they 'feel' would be the right treatment for them; often people have a 'hunch' or 'feeling' that this or that treatment would help them or their family, much as we may have a hunch or feeling that we should go to this or that shop to buy our new pair of shoes or whatever. But nobody should imagine that herbal medicine is necessarily the right choice of medicine for every single person.

3   'I Feel So Much Better'

W hen under a herbal medicine treatment patients very often use phrases such as 'I feel so much better in myself'. This frequently happens after only two or three days of treatment. Unfortunately, doctors have been known to make disparaging comments about these subjective response by patients, using such expressions as for instance: 'Well, if you think you're feeling better, then it's probably not doing you any harm'. Or: 'You're only getting better because you think you're feeling better', implying some sort of placebo effect, where the patient gets better because they believe they have been given something that works. (Incidentally, if the mind is this capable of healing the body maybe we should all be using hypnotherapy or other forms of positive suggestion on ourselves!)

In fact, however, this reporting of a feeling of well-being by patients taking herbal medicine treatment is something that should not be minimized, neither should it be dismissed as something in people's imagination that could be having a placebo effect. It is actually the result of the organs in the body beginning to work better, therefore the patients naturally feel better in themselves, in the same way that anyone with healthy organs feels well in themselves, both physically *and* emotionally.

We should always remember that the whole person is composed of both physical and non-physical aspects, and both of these aspects are involved in a state of true well-being.

4   Healing the Body

I n orthodox or drug medicine the emphasis is all on the *drug* as the agent that gives back a state of health, although it is an artificial or pseudo-state since the body did not achieve it naturally: the doctor diagnoses, and the drug prescribed for this diagnosis does the work *for* the patient's body: there is little element of change by the patient, or of learning what caused ill-health, going on in this situation: we may in fact wonder what it is that the doctor is teaching the patient, since the word 'doctor' in Latin means 'teacher'.

In herbal medicine the emphasis is on the healing of the patient's *own* body, on learning about ill-health and therefore about well-being, helped by the role of the practitioner acting more as a coach, health instructor, or perhaps 'doctor' in the true sense of the word.

5   'Normal' Health/Ill-health

' I f you're well, you can't be ill'. This adage is self-evident when we analyse it, but it is amazing how many people think it is possible to be ill if you are well. What this means is that if our health is really good, we will not acquire any illness. I would ask you to think about this for yourself.

Another saying that people often come up with goes something like: 'That's quite normal though, isn't it' in reference to their headaches, or sore throats, or pre-menstrual moods, or arthritis, or whatever common complaint they may suffer with. This is actually a mis-use of the word 'normal', and is really accepting what are very *common* complaints as inevitable or what the person calls 'normal'. We really should use the word 'common' instead of 'normal' in this respect: normal does *not* mean the standard which the majority of people have; it actually means that which is attainable by any individual, given that each person will have a different level of optimum health that is attainable for them. The best standard of health that can be achieved by an individual is what is 'normal' for that person. Just because many people suffer poor health does not mean we have to accept poor health as a 'normal' thing.

The same manner of thinking should apply as we get older. We do not need to think that it is normal to have arthritis or any other complaint as we get older. Many people do, certainly, so it is very common, but that is because their health is not as good as it might be, and poor health is not something we should accept just because we are getting older and because it is very common. Once again, we cannot be ill if we are well.

This is not to say that human health is like a horizontal line with a line somewhere about half-way along, on one side of which is a 'good' state called health, and on the other side of which is a 'bad' state called illness. Rather it is more like a thermometer in a vertical direction, with no limit as to how high the reading may go: the higher it goes, the better our health.

There is no fixed point on the scale, at which a person begins to have good health and below which she or he has poor health: the indicator on the thermometer is entirely flexible and goes up and down in response to the many factors which make up health, and there is no limit as to how far up the scale it may go.

Who is absolutely as healthy as she or he could possibly be? There is always room for an improvement in health for each of us, and always a possibility that the health can rise up the scale if the right measures are taken.

6   Listening to the Patient

S omething that patients have said consistently to the author over his years in practice is how gratifying it is to be listened to by a medical practitioner. Doctors, he has been told, are all too ready to tell patients what is wrong with them, rather than listening to the patient to tell them. Self-evidently, there is no-one who knows their own body better than the patient; she or he may not know the exact medical expressions to use or the exact details of physiology, but there is no-one better able to describe the symptoms being suffered, and therefore no-one better to listen to than patients themselves for a description of the illness being experienced.

7   Sustaining Plant Medicines

A major issue at the present time and in the immediate future has to be the sustainability of plant medicines: it is no good there being an explosion in the the use of herbal medicines if there are not enough plants being grown for this purpose, and we do not have a right to expect that nature will provide an unlimited amount of plants for us without our careful stewardship of them in return.

Herbalists would like to see the public who are using herbal medicines in ever-greater volumes from health food shops and other outlets, putting pressure on their suppliers to ensure that the source of the plants is known by the supplier to be a sustainable one, and that plants are not being harvested and destroyed in their wild habitats for the purpose. There are currently a number of endangered plant medicines including False Unicorn Root and Golden Seal Root: but really this principle needs to be applied to all plant medicines.

8 Echinacea

There is more to having a good immune system than just taking the herb Echinacea: in fact, a herbalist has at her or his disposal many different herbs to help the person's own immunity to strengthen itself, and chooses them according to the individual case. Echinacea cannot be expected to build someone's immunity up regardless of what is happening in the rest of their body, and regardless of what else they may be doing which may be harming or reducing their immunity.

In fact, though, many people do use Echinacea with great success. Frequently, they are unsure about how much to take or how long to take it for, however.

The popularity of Echinacea, as also of St John's Wort, raises a question of concern to herbalists and those interested in the environment and in conservation: are herbs being harvested indiscriminately in the wild and with little concern for their future availability? Do all the people taking St John's Wort know the source of their supply? Is it a sustainable one? Do they even care whether it is sustainable or not? In the case of Echinacea it is mainly the root that is used medicinally, so the plant itself may well be destroyed unless the producer is sensitive to the issue of sustainability.

9 How Herbs Work

Herbalists are often asked how herbs work. The answer is that they 'target' or have an affinity for certain organs in the body. For example, dandelion targets the liver and the kidneys. Certain herbs increase the function of these organs, and others decrease the function. The herbalist's job is to assess which organs need their function changing, that is either increasing or decreasing, and then select appropriate herbs for that individual patient's need.

Progress is then monitored and the prescription changed as the patient's condition moves on. This is the reason why there is no particular herb for high blood pressure, or psoriasis, or migraines, it depends entirely on what organic function is causing the high blood pressure, or psoriasis, or migraines in that particular person at that particular time.

FURTHER READING

Andrew Chevallier, FNIMH — *The Encyclopedia of Medicinal Plants*, London, Dorling Kindersley, 1996

Nalda Gosling, MNIMH — *Successful Herbal Remedies*, London, Thorsons, 1989

David Hoffman, MNIMH — *The New Holistic Herbal*, Element Books, 1991

Anne McIntyre, MNIMH — *The Complete Woman's Herbal*, Gaia Books, 1994

Christopher Robbins, MNIMH — *Introductory Guide to Herbalism*, London, Thorsons, 1984

Graeme Tobyn, MNIMH — *Culpeper's Medicine: A Practice of Western Holistic Medicine*, Element Books, 1997

Appendix
• • • • •

How to Find a Herbalist

UK & Europe

The National Institute of Medical Herbalists publishes a Register of Qualified Members (nearly 1000), which is available on request by sending a SAE for 100gm postage to:

> Honorary General Secretary
> The National Institute of Medical Herbalists
> 56 Longbrook Street
> Exeter
> Devon EX4 6AH
> Tel.: (01392) 426022
> Website: www.btinternet.com/~nimh

The institute also has members in Denmark, Eire, France, Germany, Iceland, Norway, Spain and Turkey, as well as many other parts of the world. Members can be identified by the letters MNIMH or FNIMH after their name.

Europe

There is a European Herbal Practitioners Association (EHPA) which is an umbrella organization comprising several different herbal registers representing the Western, Chinese and Ayurvedic traditions of herbal medicine. The EHPA is currently lobbying for appropriate European legislation for herbal medicines and is working towards the state registration of herbal practitioners throughout the EU. This process is well under way in the UK and in its initial stages in Ireland and in some other EU Member States.

The EHPA can be contacted via:

> Michael McIntyre
> Midsummer Cottage Clinic
> Nether Westcote
> Chipping Norton
> Oxon OX7 6SD
> Tel.: (01993) 830419

USA

The American Herbalists Guild is the only association of medical herbalists in the United States whose professional members are determined by an admissions review process. The Guild has specific continuing education requirements and a code of ethics. [The AHG should not be confused with the National Certification Council for Acupuncturists and Oriental Medicine (NCCAOM) which administers an annual certification test specifically for practitioners of traditional Chinese medicine (TCM).] Members of the American Herbalists Guild can be identified by the term 'Herbalists AHG'. Details from:

> American Herbalists Guild
> PO Box 70, Rosevelt, UT 84066
> Phone: (435) 722-8434   Fax: (435) 722-8452
> E-mail: ahgoffice@earthlink.net
> website: www.healthy.net/herbalists/Finding.htm

There are members of the UK's National Institute of Medical Herbalists in both the USA and Canada.

Australia and New Zealand

The UK's National Institute of Medical Herbalists also has members in Australia and New Zealand. In addition, there is the National Herbalists Association of Australia at:

> National Herbalists Association
> PO Box 61
> Broadway
> NSW 2007

Index
•••••